DUC-IT-UP!

366

TIPS

to improve your life

Sheryl,
For your journey!

Duc C. Vuong

Cover design and interior layout by Tony Loton of LOTONtech Limited.

For my father,

Phuoc Sanh Vuong,

whose courage to leave his homeland and family

is what provided me with this life

I so cherish.

A Message from Dr. V...

I cannot express how happy I am that you purchased this book. Personally, I've always wanted a book that would not only serve as my daily journal but also enrich my life. Why? I own several blank journals and have always found it difficult to stare at those blank pages every morning, knowing I'm supposed to write something monumental but couldn't. So I created this book as much for me as for you.

Each date starts with a great tip, then is followed by a poignant quote, and ends with a commitment to action. You can read it from the beginning to the end or skip to the current date. Either is fine. I hope you find one golden nugget that will help you live a better life.

This book is also meant to be a journal. You can write your long term goals as well as set your daily to do's. I've left room at the bottom for notes and ideas that might have been inspired by the passage. Try to develop a routine where you will jot down a few thoughts at the bottom, even if you think they are silly. You never know, when looking back, those "silly" ideas might strike a chord with you. If you run out of room, then please feel free to continue the writing from one page to the next. In this way, your moments of inspiration will not be limited by space. In other words, the lines at the bottom are for you to use as you wish. They do not have to be limited to the tip or even words for that matter.

If you are already not connected with me on social media, I hope you will friend me on Facebook, Periscope, Twitter, or Instagram @DrDucVuong. I also speak frequently at conferences, so I hope to meet you in person someday.

Remember, our time on this planet is quite brief. We only journey around the sun on this round rock but a few times. So let's make it a great trip.

With love,

Dr. V

January

Don't Get Distracted

"The goal is to keep the goal the goal." – Dan John

To-Do's
✔
✔
✔
✔
✔
✔
✔
✔
✔
✔

Long-Term Goals
☐
☐
☐
☐
☐
☐
☐
☐
☐
☐

Setting goals is easy. Most of us know what we want, whether it's to lose fat, get more sleep, build muscle, reduce stress, write a novel, win a gardening competition, et cetera.

Reaching the goals isn't always as easy as setting them, but nothing complicates the situation like getting derailed by distractions. For instance, imagine that someone finds a muscle building program, puts in four dedicated weeks, sees wonderful results, and then changes course entirely once he reads or hears about another program that's supposedly better. **He stops doing what is obviously working to try something that *might* work better.** Maybe it does. Or...maybe he has to backtrack and get back to basics.

Focus. Figure out your goals, choose a path, and keep going until there's a reason to change what's working. Tune out the noise as long as you're seeing results that make you happy and healthy.

Commitment: Decide not to get derailed by distractions. Watch this brief video on goal setting and maintenance from Dan John:

https://www.youtube.com/watch?v=fmGRH4eSSAs

Journal...

_____
_____
_____
_____
_____
_____
_____
_____
_____
_____
_____
_____
_____
_____
_____
_____
_____
_____
_____

Get Enough Sleep

"I love sleep. My life has a tendency to fall apart when I'm awake." – Ernest Hemingway

✓ Contact Stovall

✓

✓

✓

✓

✓

✓

✓

✓

2017

Because today is January 2, you might still be recovering from a couple of wild nights, which means you might currently be extremely familiar with what the lack of sleep feels like.

Not getting enough sleep can make you irritable. Trust me I know firsthand—as a surgical resident, I was often sleep deprived. Your brain works more sluggishly, and your energy plummets. Lack of sleep impedes fat loss, reduces the pep needed for exercise...on and on and on. There's no upside to insufficient sleep. Good luck finding part of your life that is *not* impacted by insufficient sleep. Camille Peri adds "lack of sex drive," "forgetfulness," "increased potential for depression," as well as other depressing side effects. (*10 Things To Hate About Sleep Loss, WebMD*)

You need energy, alertness, and **you *deserve* to feel as well as possible, every day.** Sleep is the core. There are a lot of things you can fight through and get away with for a long time, but not sleeping is not one of them.

Commitment: Read *No More Sleepless Nights* by Peter Hauri. Be honest about your sleep habits. Make the changes that will let you get as much sleep as you should.

☐ Be HEALTHY

☐ eAT right, do what I can to Avoid alz

☐ Build muscle

☐ do something about my obsession w/ B

☐

☐

☐

☐

Journal...

It is 11:12pm- past my bedtime- doing last minute things to get ready for bed to get ready for tomorrow - Always in a Rush trying to get many things done at once. that does not work - by focusing on 1 thing at a time - I really get more done and I am calmer. I am not drinking alot of water yet I am having "urge" and leak problems. my fat/ lack of movement has caught up to me, I'm already behind with suggestions for yesterday + Today, Go to sleep SLJ!

Eat the Appropriate Amount of Protein

"Calories from protein affect your brain, your appetite control center, so you are more satiated and satisfied." –
Dr. Mark Hyman

To-Do's		Long-Term Goals
✔	Simply put, you are made of protein. Without protein, there is no you. You'd lose your tendons, muscles, skin, organs, and more. It's not just the muscle men guzzling down protein shakes who need to be committed to their protein intake. **But you need to consume the proper amount of protein.**	☐
✔		☐
✔	Animals get enough protein because they don't have the option to choose their meals. They just eat what they eat and they get enough, assuming that food sources are available.	☐
✔		☐
✔	Daniel Pendick, former Executive Editor of Harvard Men's Health Watch, states that The Recommended Dietary Allowance (RDA) for protein is a modest 0.8 grams of protein per kilogram of body weight. (*2015, How Much Protein Do You Really Need? Harvard Medical School*). There are exceptions, of course. A male bodybuilder whose only goal is increased muscularity will require more protein for his goals. The more active we are, the more protein we need to build our bodies and replenish our protein stores.	☐
✔		☐
✔		☐
✔		☐
✔	It all varies and we're all different. But for most of us, the RDA's recommendation of .8 per kilogram of bodyweight is a good starting point. Let's assume you are a 5'5" woman and weigh 150 pounds or 67.5 kg. Therefore, your daily protein requirement is only 54 grams.	☐
✔		☐
✔		☐
✔	**Commitment:** Start tracking your protein intake in a food journal. If you are ever eating a meal without protein, add it. Shoot for the .8 grams per kilogram of bodyweight, and adjust accordingly, based on your goals and results.	☐

Journal...

_____
_____
_____
_____
_____
_____
_____
_____
_____
_____
_____
_____

Eat Lean Protein First

"One cannot think well, love well, sleep well, if one has not dined well." —Virginia Woolf

To-Do's		Long-Term Goals

✔

✔

✔

✔

✔

✔

✔

✔

If you are feeling full by the time you get to the protein on your plate, you might not be able to finish it. If you're trying to increase your protein intake, this causes a conundrum. You could choke down the rest of the protein on your plate and cause yourself some intestinal distress and regret, or you could try something simpler.

Just eat the protein first. You will get full faster, and ensure that your protein requirements are met, assuming you've got some protein on your plate, as you now know you should. Protein releases the peptide Ghrelin, which is known as the "hunger hormone." Protein (via Ghrelin) literally satiates you faster than other food sources. It's why you can eat three pounds of rice and still feel hungry, but a modest size portion of fish can make you feel full before you're even finished. I recommend that my patients **choose leaner sources of protein**, such as beans, whole grains, lentils, tofu, fish, and seafood.

Commitment: Make sure there's some lean protein on your plate. Then, eat it first. You'll be more satisfied and you won't be able to eat as much.

☐ ☐ ☐ ☐ ☐ ☐ ☐ ☐

Journal...

_____
_____
_____
_____
_____
_____
_____
_____
_____
_____
_____
_____
_____
_____
_____
_____
_____
_____
_____
_____
_____
_____
_____

Learn Gym Etiquette

"Etiquette means behaving yourself a little better than is absolutely essential."—Will Cuppy

To-Do's		Long-Term Goals

Developing a regular gym-going habit can be tough, but there are things that can make it harder. Namely, the other people in the gym. Most are considerate, many are not. Gym etiquette is not hard to learn, and it will make sure that you're never an annoying part of someone else's gym experience.

First and foremost, if you use a weight, put it back. Easy. Next, if you use a machine and leave sweat on it, any visible sweat at all, wipe it off. Most gyms have paper towel dispensers and disinfectant sprays. Also, there's no need to scream and beat your chest while you're lifting. Nobody should have any reason to turn up their headphones to drown you out.

A couple more. There are exceptions, but the gym is not a social club. Lots of people are there to *work*. Don't interrupt them by hitting on them or offering unsolicited advice. Let people do their thing. If they're sending out signals, you'll know. If they don't, again, let them do their thing.

Commitment: Quick and easy, right? Learn basic gym etiquette and practice it.

Journal...

Sit Less

"Scientists have determined that after an hour or more of sitting, the production of enzymes that burn fat in the body declines by as much as 90 percent" – The New York Times, Taking a Stand for Office Ergonomics

To-Do's		Long-Term Goals
✔	If you're like most people, you spend a lot of time sitting. Unless you have a physical job demanding that you stoop, stretch, lift, carry, and twist, you probably spend the majority of your day in front of a computer or pushing papers. Chances are, that means you're in a chair.	☐
✔		☐
✔	Now, if you spend most of your life in a chair, you're eventually going to be shaped like a chair! **Your body is always going to try to assume the position that you make it spend most of its time in.** The good news is that you can always find a way to put your body in a more optimal position. Correcting the influence of the omnipresent chairs in our lives will take some dedication, but very little effort. You just have to commit to better habits.	☐
✔		☐
✔		☐
✔		☐
✔	**Commitment:** While sitting, sit up straight, shoulders back, and move to the front of the seat. Stand up and move for one minute out of every 30. Walk around. Shake your arms out. Rotate your wrists in both directions so they're not always in "typing" position. Get creative and do the opposite of what sitting in a chair looks like. Consider sitting on a bouncy core ball instead of a chair.	☐
✔		☐
✔		☐

Journal...

_____
_____
_____
_____
_____
_____
_____
_____
_____
_____
_____
_____
_____
_____
_____
_____
_____
_____
_____
_____
_____

Move More

"All motion is cyclic. It circulates to the limits of its possibilities and then returns to its starting point." – Robert Collier

To-Do's		Long-Term Goals

A body in balance can perform any of the big movement patterns without distress. Squatting, pushing horizontally or vertically, pulling horizontally or vertically, lifting things from the floor, crawling, skipping, and so on. **When there is a movement pattern that makes you groan, this is a sign that mobility has been lost.**

We already ditched the chair in the previous tip, but now we have to get ourselves moving more. The culprit in so many cases of lingering pain and poor posture is our increasingly sedentary lifestyle.

Here is a gentle starting point to start recapturing and strengthening any movement patterns you may have lost. You don't even need to use weight in order to reap the benefit of a movement like the squat. Just take your body through the movement of squatting down and standing back up. Do it without pain, and don't go nuts with a million repetitions. We're just trying to reintroduce movements that will keep us healthier over the long term.

Commitment: Perform each of the movement patterns, as long as you are not in pain, each day. Squat, vertical and horizontal push (think of the pushup motion or pressing weight overhead), vertical and horizontal pull (think pullups or "rowing" weight towards yourself like an oar), and lifting things off the floor, whether it's a loaded barbell or a basket of laundry. Just make sure they're all in the rotation.

Journal...

_____
_____
_____
_____
_____
_____
_____
_____
_____
_____
_____
_____
_____
_____
_____
_____

January 8

Smile More

"If you smile when no one else is around, you really mean it." – Andy Rooney

To-Do's

- ✔
- ✔
- ✔
- ✔
- ✔
- ✔

Long-Term Goals

- ☐
- ☐
- ☐
- ☐
- ☐
- ☐

If you know how good it feels to be smiled at, you know the power of a smile. If you never feel like smiling, then you're missing out on some amazing benefits. A 2012 study by University of Kansas Psychological Scientists found that smiling reduced the heart rate and shortened the time needed to recover from stressful situations. (*Kraft and Pressman, Grin and Bear It, Psychological Science, 2012*).

But we all know that smiling just feels *good,* as long as we have something to smile about. And that, of course, is just one more reason to **fill your life with things, people, and experiences that will keep you smiling.**

Commitment: Watch yourself smile in the mirror when you don't feel like it. Pay attention to how you feel. Today commit to smiling at everyone you come into contact with.

Journal...

Track Your Progress

"Today's progress was yesterday's plan." – Unknown

To-Do's		Long-Term Goals

There is nothing abstract about Progress. You're either stronger, or healthier, or more well-read, or more slender than you were the day before. It's obvious--as long as you keep track of it. This is one of the keys to long-term enthusiasm for our goals. Everything that is measurable, can be tracked. **What you can track, you can improve.**

Regardless of your goal, a progress log can be invaluable. If you're always keeping track of your progress, you never have to guess about what you should do today, whether it's the next workout, how many miles you should run, how many words you need to add to your book or blog, and so on.

This can also lead to a huge increase in confidence. If you are always improving at something, and you can *see* it happening in your progress log, you will *feel* more confident. How could you not?

Tracking your progress helps eliminate the guesswork for you. Because if you're guessing, there's always the chance that you'll guess incorrectly.

Commitment: Find a measurable goal, like lose 10 pounds in 2 months or increase your savings by $500 in one month. Track your goals in a journal. Record all progress, adjust according to your results, and celebrate every achievement.

Journal...

_____
_____
_____
_____
_____
_____
_____
_____
_____
_____
_____
_____
_____
_____
_____
_____
_____
_____
_____

Read!

*"The more that you read, the more things you will know. The more that you learn, the more places you'll go." –
Dr. Seuss, I Can Read With My Eyes Shut!*

To-Do's

✔

✔

✔

✔

✔

✔

✔

✔

Reading flexes parts of your brain that nothing else will. It's really a marvel when you think about it. Everything that has ever been written in English was done with only 26 letters. But the process by which our brain takes apart those little squiggles of ink on the pages or the pixels on the screen is anything but simple.

Reading requires innumerable acts of mental computation that keep the brain firing. It also enhances our ability to think analytically and engage with complex arguments, a skill that is being diminished in the click-happy age of instant gratification on the internet.

I don't just mean books. Read regularly, and then **read outside of your comfort zone.**

Commitment: Take time to read every day, even if it's just one page. Once you're in the habit, go outside of your comfort zone. If you usually read fiction, try self-help. If you usually read books, read an essay. If you're always reading essays, try historical autobiographies. The options are endless. Stretch and grow.

Long-Term Goals

☐

☐

☐

☐

☐

☐

☐

☐

Journal...

_____
_____
_____
_____
_____
_____
_____
_____
_____
_____
_____
_____
_____
_____
_____
_____
_____
_____
_____
_____
_____
_____

Go For a Walk

"I don't know what my path is yet. I'm just walking on it." – Olivia Newton John

To-Do's		Long-Term Goals

We are rarely required to walk very far. You drive yourself to work, then you sit at the computer, then you drive yourself home, then you relax on the couch, then you slumber in bed for eight hours. Just to repeat the process the next day. Think about how rarely you need to perform the simple act of putting one foot in front of the other.

Walks, however long, seem to inspire reflection and contemplation. They can help restore mobility, strengthen our cardiovascular systems, and provide a way to see more of the world.

Walking causes us to focus on our surroundings, which can help with the practice of mindfulness. There are monks whose entire meditation practice is comprised of short walks and intense thought. Even if the ascetic element of walking doesn't appeal to you, the tranquility of a self-imposed leisurely stroll will.

Commitment: Get in 10,000 steps today. Then walk for a mile, three times a week. Focus on your surroundings and try to contemplate the steps, as your foot strikes the ground. Increase the distance or the frequency next week

Journal...

Eat Organic When Possible

"You are what what you eat eats." – Michael Pollan

To-Do's
✔
✔
✔
✔
✔
✔
✔
✔
✔
✔

Long-Term Goals
☐
☐
☐
☐
☐
☐
☐
☐
☐
☐

Scenario: Can I get you to eat this giant, scrumptious bowl of pesticides and weird chemicals? Wait! Where are you going? I've got tomatoes, basil, beef, corn, avocados, and *all* of it is probably contaminated with contaminants you should never put in your body!

Of course, you'd never willing do this. But you can buy these tainted foods at your local grocer. Buying organic doesn't eliminate all possibility of encountering unwanted chemicals, but it increases the odds dramatically. It is as healthy as possible for many of us to eat, short of growing our own food.

It's an old joke at this point. "Shop at Whole Foods? More like Whole Paycheck! Ha!" It is true that buying organic can cost more, financially. **But when it comes to your health, is it truly expensive?** Are you being reckless by spending a few extra dollars in order to increase your current well-being and long-term health? If you can't see the health benefits, then I ask, isn't it worth spending a few extra dollars to stop poisoning your family?

Commitment: Buy organic as often as possible. It certainly doesn't need to be from Whole Foods, but seek out the organic labels in the store of your choice. Learn more about the most contaminated foods, such as strawberries, thereby, maximizing the benefit of buying organic.

Journal...

_____
_____
_____
_____
_____
_____
_____
_____
_____
_____
_____
_____
_____
_____
_____
_____
_____
_____
_____

Find the Right Shoes

"I did not have three thousand pairs of shoes, I had one thousand and sixty." – Imelda Marcos

To-Do's		Long-Term Goals

Think about the job our feet have. These two little planks, made of such tiny delicate bones, have to support our weight and carry us around, year after year. They do this whether they're arched, flat, covered in bunions, or sore. How many steps do you think you take in a day? A year? A lifetime? **Your feet carry you every single time you take a step.**

Treating them right is a good decision. When you start to experience foot pain, you'll adjust your gait accordingly. Adjusting your stride can lead to your feet pointing outward or inward, walking on your heels instead of putting more weight on the balls of your feet, walking on the outside of your feet if your instep is agitated, and so on into near infinite variations.

Get comfortable shoes and replace them as often as you need to. Treat your feet as if you're grateful for the beasts of burden that they are.

Commitment: Read *Born to Run* by Christopher McDougall. It's a fascinating book about a South American tribe whose culture revolves around running, and an insightful study of the evolution of our feet.

Journal...

Get More Probiotics

"Most bacteria aren't bad. We breathe and eat and ingest gobs of bacteria every single moment of our lives. Our food is covered in bacteria. And you're breathing in bacteria all the time, and you mostly don't get sick." –
Bonnie Bassler

To-Do's
✔
✔
✔
✔
✔
✔
✔
✔
✔
✔

With the possible exception of migraine headaches and toothaches, few discomforts are as hard to ignore as intestinal distress. If you deal with chronic digestive problems, or you just think you might be able to feel better than you do, probiotics could be a good start.

Essentially, probiotics move food through your gut. **Probiotics are good bacteria.** Now, bacteria is a word that often makes people flinch. It might be hard to imagine that you'd ever want bacteria inside of you--not that you can help it. Probiotics can help fight the bad bacteria, or keep them in balance. It's really not so different from building up an immunity to a virus through a vaccination.

It's time to let go of the negative connotations tied to the word. No doctor would ask you to down a cup of a harmful bacteria just for fun, but all would agree that something as simple as a cup of yogurt--filled with probiotics, incidentally--can work wonders to balance the good bacteria with the bad.

Commitment: Get more probiotics. Yogurt, soft cheeses, and probiotic supplements are all easy places to start.

Long-Term Goals
☐
☐
☐
☐
☐
☐
☐
☐

Journal...

_____
_____
_____
_____
_____
_____
_____
_____
_____
_____
_____
_____
_____
_____
_____
_____
_____
_____
_____
_____
_____

20/20/20 Blinking

"Vision is the art of seeing what is invisible to others." – Jonathan Swift

To-Do's		Long-Term Goals

Like the rest of our bodies, our eyes age. But there are few things that feel as bad as irritated, dry, fuzzy eyes. The amount of time many of us spend looking at electronic screens isn't helping. It's easy to forget to blink when on a computer. You might get more done, but you'll pay a price.

Here is a simple solution that I got from an optometrist, and that has worked wonders for me. Every 20 minutes, look at an object 20 feet away--something featureless, like a blank section of wall is preferable--and blink 20 times, slightly pressing your eyelids together each time. This isn't rapid fire blinking. It's meant to **lubricate your eyes.** The firmer and longer you can make each blink, the better your eyes will feel afterward.

It is much more likely that you can stick to this routine than that all the electronic screens will suddenly vanish from your life.

Commitment: Practice 20/20/20 blinking and read Dr. Robert Joyce's article on Huffington Post: *Overworked eyes: Will Your Computer Make You Go Blind?*

http://www.huffingtonpost.com/robert-joyce-od/eye-strain_b_1591414.html

Journal...

Use a Neti Pot

Ruth: "Where do you keep your... nostril pot?"
George: "Neti pot."
Six Feet Under: Terror Starts At Home

To-Do's

- ✔
- ✔
- ✔
- ✔
- ✔
- ✔
- ✔

Whether it's cold season or not, the sinus cavities can be a repository of germs and dryness that can drive you nuts. But how to clean it out? There aren't many options for flushing it out.

Enter the neti pot, an ancient remedy that many people in America first heard of on the HBO show *Six Feet Under*. You fill a pot—most are about the size of a small teapot—fill it with a mix of water and saline solution, or salt, and put one end in your nose.

Then you tilt your head over a sink and gently pour it through one nostril. It irrigates the channel and comes out the other nostril. It's not the most tasteful sounding thing in the world, but your sinuses—and your resistance to colds—will thank you.

Commitment: Give it a try. Neti pots are inexpensive and can be found in nearly any store with a pharmacy.

Long-Term Goals

- ☐
- ☐
- ☐
- ☐
- ☐
- ☐
- ☐

Journal...

Travel More

"Travel is fatal to prejudice, bigotry, and narrow-mindedness." – Mark Twain

To-Do's		Long-Term Goals

To-Do's
- ✔
- ✔
- ✔
- ✔
- ✔
- ✔
- ✔
- ✔
- ✔
- ✔

If you're not happy with yourself, simply going to a different might be just what you need. Few things expand your horizons like travel.

Travel is a way to see new things, new people, new customs, and to gain a greater appreciation for our own homes and lives. In fact, it's impossible to travel and *not* experience newness. No matter your situation, your perspective is necessarily limited by how much of the world you have seen.

And this might sound like a ridiculously obvious thing to say, but travel can make you appreciate your own home more. Few things feel as nice as coming back to your space, even after a wonderful trip. But you can't come home without leaving.

Incidentally, one of the definitions of the word "adventure" is "undetermined outcome." You never know what you'll get when you head somewhere new, which can be a brilliant thing.

Commitment: Take a short road trip this upcoming weekend with your loved one. Also plan an extended vacation this year, and make sure it's somewhere you have never been.

Long-Term Goals
- ☐
- ☐
- ☐
- ☐
- ☐
- ☐
- ☐
- ☐
- ☐
- ☐

Journal...

_____
_____
_____
_____
_____
_____
_____
_____
_____
_____
_____
_____
_____
_____
_____
_____
_____
_____
_____
_____

Try a Tongue Scraper

"There's always a germ of truth in just about everything." – Jim Lehrer

To-Do's
✔
✔
✔
✔
✔
✔
✔
✔
✔

Long-Term Goals
☐
☐
☐
☐
☐
☐
☐
☐
☐

Okay, so maybe Jim Lehrer's quote doesn't mean that the germs in our mouths are germs of truth, but there's no disputing that our mouths are veritable playgrounds for germs, bacteria, and toxins. Between eating, chewing, breathing, and all of the other tasks our mouths are given, there is a lot going on in there.

The mouth is the primary way foreign bacteria and viruses enter the body. Even though the tongue is wet and constantly lubricated, it's still a magnet for bacterial toxins. Toxins don't just wash off because our tongues live in a moist environment. Those that linger on the tongue can be absorbed into the body. At that point it's going to be tougher to rid our bodies of them. So, what to do?

Invest in a tongue scraper. It's exactly what it sounds like. After brushing your teeth, you run a tongue scraper over your tongue a couple of times. The amount of gunk you'll see might shock you, but it will certainly help you see that a daily scraping is going to spare your body some unpleasantness.

Commitment: Buy a tongue scraper and use it daily. They're cheap and it only takes a few seconds to use. This practice has been used in Asian cultures for centuries.

Journal...

_____
_____
_____
_____
_____
_____
_____
_____
_____
_____
_____
_____
_____
_____
_____
_____
_____
_____
_____
_____
_____

Don't Grocery Shop When You're Hungry

"I love grocery shopping...that's what makes me feel totally normal." – Yo-Yo Ma

To-Do's		Long-Term Goals

✔

✔

✔

✔

✔

✔

✔

✔

When you are hungry, a trip to the grocery store can make you feel like a dusty traveler stumbling out of the desert, collapsing at the edge of an oasis, and slurping down the water until you're sick to your stomach.

Have you ever looked down at your shopping cart and seen an astonishing amount of food? Or worse, an abundance of snacks that you've been craving? **Hunger can make us impulsive**, and we might treat the simple act of grocery shopping as if it's the last time we'll ever have a chance to eat. And, again, the foods we crave often seem to make frequent appearances during these shopping trips of imaginary desperation.

Whenever possible, enter the grocery store with a satisfied stomach that isn't nagging you. You'll be more clear-headed and shop like someone who needs groceries, not a binge-happy lunatic.

Commitment: Eat something before you go to the store. Preferably with protein which will work as an appetite suppressant. A handful of raw almonds would be great.

☐ ☐ ☐ ☐ ☐ ☐ ☐ ☐

Journal...

Cut Back On Alcohol

"That's all drugs and alcohol do, they cut off your emotions in the end." – Ringo Starr

To-Do's		Long-Term Goals

✔

✔

✔

✔

✔

✔

✔

✔

✔

Alcohol can be a lot of fun. And, like most things that can be fun, it can be *too* much fun. "How much is too much?" is a question that each of us have to answer for ourselves. **But there is rarely a downside to drinking less.** And if you ever catch yourself wondering if you should drink less, the answer is probably less.

You'll feel less sluggish in the morning, if you did not drink the night before, and you might feel a lot happier. Alcohol, however lively it makes you in the moment, is a psychological depressant.

Long-term abuse results in a host of problems, including liver failure. But you don't need to be a hardcore abuser in order to benefit from a break. And it doesn't even need to be a long break, just enough to give yourself time to reevaluate your intake and ask yourself some questions that might not occur to you if you're drinking a few times a week.

Commitment: Reduce your alcohol intake by half for a week. Observe your mood, how your body feels, and your wallet. If you like the results, consider making the commitment to reducing your drinking further still.

☐ ☐ ☐ ☐ ☐ ☐ ☐ ☐ ☐

Journal...

_____
_____
_____
_____
_____
_____
_____
_____
_____
_____
_____
_____
_____
_____
_____
_____
_____
_____
_____
_____
_____

Learn To Cook

"Cooking is like painting or writing a song. Just as there are only so many notes or colors, there are only so many flavors - it's how you combine them that sets you apart." – Wolfgang Puck

To-Do's

✔

✔

✔

✔

✔

✔

✔

✔

✔

Long-Term Goals

☐ ☐ ☐ ☐ ☐ ☐ ☐ ☐ ☐

Cooking is such an easy way to make people happy, including yourself! Everyone loves a good cook, but you don't have to turn yourself into a culinary wiz to reap the benefits of learning your way around a kitchen and stove. Think back to your college days, when you had only two bowls, one fork, and a spoon if you were really fancy—it's time to learn how to prepare a few simple meals.

The best reason is that you can control what goes into your food. If someone else prepares your food, you have to take their ingredients and abilities in good faith. Whether it's delicious or not, someone else had control over what you're eating. But if you go to the grocery store, shop for the right ingredients, and are involved in every step of the preparation, **you know exactly what you're going to put into your body**.

It can be a great way to save money, too. Eating lots of fast food is good for your wallet in the short-term, but it does add up over time. And a chronic fast-food habit is always going to be bad for your health.

Commitment: Add one simple dish to your cooking repertoire twice a month. Before long you'll be ready to impress.

Journal...

Stretch

"I love stretching in the morning. It's the first thing I do when I wake up because getting a good back-crack is so extremely satiating. I feel taller when I finally stand." – Rachel Nichols

To-Do's
✔
✔
✔
✔
✔
✔
✔

Unless you're up and moving all day, there's a very good chance that you have knots of rigid muscle tissue. If you don't take time to stretch, your tendons can actually shorten and lock you into bad postures.

For instance, have you ever seen an elderly person whose walks stooped, shoulders pulled forward, and bending at the waist? This is a person who did not spend adequate time in the opposite position, with shoulders back and hip flexors stretched. They are now tethered to this posture, and, while there is a way to fix this, **it's easiest to prevent it before it can even start.**

Your muscles can't shorten and tighten up on you if you don't let them. A few minutes a day and you'll avoid problems that are incredibly difficult to reverse in old age.

Commitment: Stretch for five minutes a day. Once you're in the habit, try a gentle yoga routine for beginners next month.

Long-Term Goals
☐
☐
☐
☐
☐
☐
☐

Journal...

_____
_____
_____
_____
_____
_____
_____
_____
_____
_____
_____
_____
_____
_____
_____
_____
_____
_____
_____
_____
_____
_____

Go Outside

"If getting our kids out into nature is a search for perfection, or is one more chore, then the belief in perfection and the chore defeats the joy. It's a good thing to learn more about nature in order to share this knowledge with children; it's even better if the adult and child learn about nature together. And it's a lot more fun." –
Richard Louv

To-Do's

- ✓
- ✓
- ✓
- ✓
- ✓
- ✓
- ✓
- ✓
- ✓

Long-Term Goals

- ☐
- ☐
- ☐
- ☐
- ☐
- ☐
- ☐
- ☐
- ☐

Real life does not happen online. Okay, some of it does, but there is a world beyond the computer screen. But this can be easy to forget when a smartphone or computer gives you the sensation that you're *everywhere at once* and that everything is available to you.

But your smartphone does not give you fresh air to breathe. It may not induce a tranquil state as you click on link after link and scan article after article. **Looking at a picture of a sunrise or sunset does not give you the feel of the sun on your skin.** Even in the midst of winter, the chill in the air might be what we need to shock our system back into the present moment.

Going outside doesn't necessarily have to mean it's time for you to commune with nature, although there's nothing wrong with that. But it's important to spend some time in natural light, soak up the Vitamin D, to survive the sting of the cold air in our lungs, and feel the quiet sleep of our world in hibernation. The real world.

Commitment: Start small. Spend ten minutes outside each day. If there is snow outside, then make snow angels and build a snowman, as when you were a child. You will feel better.

Journal...

Try Yoga

"Yoga is a light, which once lit, will never dim. The better your practice, the brighter the flame." – B.K.S. Iyengar

To-Do's
✔
✔
✔
✔
✔
✔
✔
✔
✔

For some of us, yoga conjures up images of gurus in loincloths who have contorted their bodies into positions that are the stuff of circus performances. But the practice of yoga can be as simple--and easy--as the practitioner chooses.

Yoga will make you more flexible and help you ease back into movement patterns you may have lost. It can strengthen your core and teach you to pay attention to your breathing, which will make your other areas of mindfulness practice more fruitful. It can tone your muscles and leave you happily tired in a way that will help you sleep deeper.

The key is simply that you try. *Any* yoga will give you the effects that anyone reaps from it, as long as you are always striving to go a little further, to hold a pose a little longer, and to pay attention to how your body and mind respond. **Yoga means "union."** And its practice is designed to get you reconnected to your true energies.

Commitment: Find a simple yoga routine you enjoy and adhere to it for one week. Start with a YouTube channel or home DVD set. Pay attention to the results. Then join a yoga studio near your home.

Long-Term Goals
☐
☐
☐
☐
☐
☐
☐
☐
☐

Journal...

_____
_____
_____
_____
_____
_____
_____
_____
_____
_____
_____
_____
_____
_____
_____
_____
_____
_____
_____
_____

Do Something You Love

"My mission in life is not merely to survive, but to thrive; and to do so with some passion, some compassion, some humor, and some style."—Maya Angelou

To-Do's		Long-Term Goals

Lots of people confuse living a passionate life with having a favorite TV show. Do you have something you are *truly* passionate about? Next question: how often do you take time to do it? Next question: If you don't have a passion, how would you go about finding one? The answer often lies in the past, where you almost certainly had something you would have dropped everything to indulge in.

It could be playing the piano, or reading short stories. It could be knitting, or riding a motorcycle, or going to the movies with friends. Too many people let their hobbies go as adult life and the working world converge. But, even if you're a master at meeting your obligations to everyone else, **don't forget that you must also meet your obligations to yourself.** Don't forget that you are living *your* life. And a surefire way to slow down your life and give it meaning specifically for yourself is to ensure that you make time for your passions.

Commitment: If you have something you love and you're not doing it, make time for it today. Open up the guitar case. Dust off the journal of your poetry. Pick up the paint brushes. If you don't have anything, find a hobby. If you can't come up with one, look to your past for clues.

Journal...

Get Involved In Your Community

"One can acquire everything in solitude except character."—Stendahl

To-Do's		Long-Term Goals

Nothing can feel as isolating as the feeling of loneliness. We can't always be in a romantic relationship, not all of us have children, or families, and sometimes even friendships can be hard to come by.

But there is always a way to get involved in your community at large. There are always people who need help. **And there will be times when helping others might be the best way to help yourself.** Volunteering your time and effort to your community will inevitably guide you to a larger circle of people. That larger circle will contain people that you bond with. Those people will become a smaller community that will become your circle.

There is no better way to get out of your own misery than to serve the people around you. And because we all need help, there will never be a shortage of opportunities to serve.

Commitment: Volunteer just one hour of your time today or this weekend, for a cause you support. Then make a commitment to do more.

Journal...

Interrupt Yourself

"The first principle is that you must not fool yourself — and you are the easiest person to fool." – Richard Feynman

To-Do's		Long-Term Goals

If you nod with familiarity at this Feynman quote, you might agree that you can fool yourself into thinking that you are an awful, unlovable, lazy, dumb, irritating, and useless person.

You're not.

So many of life's ills come, not just from the negative things we tell ourselves, but from our inability to *interrupt* these internal scolding marathons. **Your own little voice is *always* there in your head.** It's not always going to say nice things and fill you with confidence.

Learning how to get a break from it can be nearly as good as eliminating it entirely. We are the only animals who can observe ourselves and recognize our moods for what they are: moods. To break this pattern of negative story-telling, find a trigger word that will alert you to stop. Any word will work, as long as you associate it with the need to stop the negative self-talk.

Commitment: When you are really laying into yourself, say out loud, "Stop." Or "Purple." Or the name of your abusive ex. Distract yourself with breathing, positive thoughts, going for a run, anything that works for you. But do not give these thoughts more importance than they deserve.

Journal...

Deal With Old Regrets

"Maybe all one can do is hope to end up with the right regrets."—Arthur Miller

To-Do's	Long-Term Goals

Regret festers like a cold sore. Even if it's not on your mind at the conscious level, regret leaves a residue that will hound you until you can truly leave it behind. And when you pile regret upon regret without ever resolving them, the accumulation of regret is far worse than any single regret.

It—and we all have our "it"—can't always be put right. If you regret the harsh words you spoke to someone you'll never see again, you'll never get to hear them say, "I forgive you." There is no going back. After your divorce, if you spend all of your time wishing you had spent more time with your family, this is futility. You *did not* do things differently.

We all *believe* that dwelling on the past *might* be useful, to the extent that it changes our future behavior. But it never actually changes the past. And the regrets involving other people are often the most painful. But they are also the regrets with the most potential for future resolution, because if you still have access to people you wish to reconcile with, there is always a chance.

Commitment: Today, reach out to someone who is involved with a past regret of yours. Do whatever you can to bring about a resolution so that you can free up that emotional headspace for yourself.

Journal...

_____
_____
_____
_____
_____
_____
_____
_____
_____
_____
_____
_____
_____
_____
_____
_____
_____
_____
_____

Keep a Journal

"I never travel without my diary. One should always have something sensational to read in the train." – Oscar Wilde

To-Do's		Long-Term Goals

When you are depressed, or when your circumstances are bad, it can be hard to remember that things were ever good. **Keeping a journal is one of the best ways to remind yourself of how good life can be.** If you write about your life every day, even if it's just a couple of sentences, you'll be able to look back and say, "Huh, I guess there are plenty of times when I had it pretty good."

Journals provide a record of perspective. They can remind us that everything passes, that there were times when we loved ourselves, and restore our hope for better days ahead.

A series of journals is also a fantastic way to let your posterity know who you were, the good and the bad. Some of the most important stories the world has would have been lost if people had not committed the simple act of writing them down.

Commitment: Get a journal and write a paragraph every day. I keep several going at all times. It can be a list of what happened, a description of how you felt, anything. Just get the words down for a month. Hopefully you've been using this book as your journal.

Journal...

January 30

Choose Kindness

"No act of kindness, no matter how small, is ever wasted." – Aesop

To-Do's		Long-Term Goals

Has there *ever* been a time when you wish you had been *less* kind? Probably not. Imagine the difference we might see if everyone on earth simply decided to be kinder to other people.

The author Kurt Vonnegut, who survived the World War II firebombing of Dresden, often said that if you went back far enough, **nearly every conflict could initially be traced back to a simple lack of kindness of courtesy.**

Try this thought experiment: What do you think would happen if everyone on earth committed to one act of kindness, every day? Most of those acts would have a positive effect on others, perhaps leading them to treat others more kindly.

We don't have any idea how far-reaching the effects would be.

Commitment: Whether it's paying for the toll fare for the car behind you or buying a stranger lunch, perform one anonymous act of kindness today. Try to do this every day.

Journal...

Breathe Before Speaking In Anger

"You will not be punished for your anger; you will be punished by your anger." – The Buddha

To-Do's		Long-Term Goals

We can't avoid the situations that will make us irritated, annoyed, agitated, angry, or flat out furious. But we can always choose our reaction.

This is not to say that anger has no place in adult life, or that it is to be avoided at all costs. Some things are worth being outraged about. In this tip, we're talking about not speaking too hastily when reacting to sudden unpleasantness. Someone says something. You want to snap back, which is natural. And this is certainly not a recommendation to avoid sticking up for yourself. But try this.

When you find yourself suddenly angry, and you're about to say something you might regret, or that might make future relationships challenging, **take a slow, deep breath.** The oxygen will help fight that constricting feeling that comes with instant negativity, it will help steady your heart rate, and most importantly, it will give you a little more time to *think before you speak.*

Commitment: The next time you feel like speaking in anger, make yourself take a long, slow breath. Count to 100. Not 10, but 100. When you're done, you may find that you are now better equipped to say whatever you need to say, thoughtfully and with greater calm.

Journal...

February

Wash Your Hands

"Normal is nothing more than a cycle on a washing machine."—Whoopi Goldberg

To-Do's		Long-Term Goals

Begin the shortest month with a clean start.

In the NPR story *The Doctor Who Championed Hand-Washing and Briefly Saved Lives*, we learn of Hungarian Physician Ignaz Semmelweis. To make a long story short—although it's well worth a listen—Semmelweis greatly reduced the number of deaths in patients under his care by instructing staff to wash their hands with chlorine.

And so the germs from the hospital staff no longer jumped from their hands into the bodies of their patients. Now, even though this was a momentous shift, there are reasons to wash your hands even if you're not a doctor. **Namely, there's no reason to subject yourself, or others, to avoidable germs.**

If you work with the public, your hands are dirty. If you use the restroom, your hands have germs on them. If you take out the garbage, ditto. They're impossible to avoid, but easy to eradicate directly after a germy task.

Commitment: This could not be more simple. Wash your hands when they have germs on them.

Journal...

Ditch the Phone (Sometimes)

"Apparently we love our own cell phones but we hate everyone else's."—Joe Bob Briggs

To-Do's		Long-Term Goals

To-Do's
- ✔
- ✔
- ✔
- ✔
- ✔
- ✔
- ✔
- ✔
- ✔

How much time do you spend looking at your phone each day? How many times a day do you *think* you look at it? I suspect the real answers would knock us for a loop. Now, our time is our own, to do with as we choose. It's your time to make the most of, and it's also your time to waste.

But there is little, in terms of wellness, to recommend when it comes to constant, compulsive smartphone use. Do we *need* to log into Facebook again, or are we doing it out of habit? Do we *need* to check on the weather, or are we just reaching for our phones instead of looking out the window because that's just what we do?

The pursuit of wellness is largely a pursuit to free ourselves from compulsions as we form better habits. If you're to the point where your phone is a compulsion, consider that it might be time for a break, or at least time to regiment your use.

Commitment: Today and tomorrow, commit to recording how many times you check your phone. Estimate that each interaction takes 30 seconds, just for a baseline. Add it up. Ask yourself if you need to be on your phone as much as you are.

Long-Term Goals
- ☐
- ☐
- ☐
- ☐
- ☐
- ☐
- ☐
- ☐
- ☐

Journal...

Breathe Deeply

"I definitely have an alter ego that can come out and get me out of situations where I'm having social anxiety. I can take a deep breath and create a bubble so I can perform in some way."—Lindy Booth

To-Do's		Long-Term Goals

The busier we are, the less likely we are to breathe deeply, regularly, and smoothly. Deep breathing—and I don't mean big, exaggerated, eyes-closed breaths that would confuse everyone around you—requires attention and a level of relaxation. **And relaxation is exactly what is missing when we're breathing shallowly.**

If you're not getting enough oxygen, you are operating at a level of mild distress, even if you're not asphyxiating. If each of your inhalations takes half a second, there's no way to pretend you're getting as much air as you could. And as a consequence, your brain is suffering.

Deep breathing is a habit that you can form consciously, and then, if you do it enough, your parasympathetic nervous system will take it from there once you teach it what to do.

Commitment: Spend two hours, regardless of what you're doing, taking slower, deeper breaths. Shoot for at least two second inhalations, and then two second exhalations. Try to fill your stomach with air, not your lungs. If your stomach is rising when you inhale, you're taking in more air than when your chest rises alone.

Journal...

Find A Mentor

"Do not train a child to learn by force or harshness; but direct them to it by what amuses their minds, so that you may be better able to discover with accuracy the peculiar bent of the genius of each." – Plato

To-Do's		Long-Term Goals

Each of us could learn something from any other person on earth. This doesn't require the person to be educated, only to be someone other than ourselves. **Experience itself is a teacher, and we can learn from the experiences of others.**

However, there is great value in a formal mentoring relationship. My life really elevated once I found a mentor. This doesn't mean you need to find a mentor and sign a contract. Only that if you have specific goals, and a specific idea of success, your mentor should be someone who has accomplished what you wish to accomplish. That person will be the most insightful teacher for you.

Before sitting down with a prospective mentor, know exactly what you hope to get out of it, and what you can offer in return.

Commitment: Find a mentor who has accomplished something that you would like to accomplish. Reach out and ask if they would be open to the possibility. The worst thing that could happen is simply that they say no, and if that occurs, you can always approach someone else.

Journal...

Be A Mentor

"No one learns as much about a subject as one who is forced to teach it." – Peter F. Drucker

To-Do's		Long-Term Goals

Once you have experienced what it is like to truly be mentored, you will become more aware that you could also be a mentor to someone else. Your experience and expertise will be valuable to someone else, and **the experience of sharing your expertise with someone else will enrich you both.** I know that has been true in my case.

Mentorship is also an exercise in encouragement. If you're a writer, you can encourage and coach an aspiring writer. If you're a physics master, you can convince a burgeoning physicist that he or she *can* get their head around the laws of nature. If your quilt wins a blue ribbon at the fair, there are probably people in your area who would love to talk quilting with you.

Commitment: Start paying attention and listening to what the people around you say they need, or want for themselves. When you find a good match, offer to be a mentor figure.

Journal...

Get A Foam Roller

"I love a massage. I'd go every day if I could. I don't need to be wrapped in herbs like a salmon fillet, but I do love a massage." – Jason Bateman

To-Do's		Long-Term Goals

If you've ever had a massage, you've probably thought "I'd love to do this more often." And then, you probably don't think of it again until you're getting another massage down the road. Massages can be expensive, and the time it takes can be prohibitive as well. If only there were a way to massage yourself and get rid of those knots.

Enter the foam roller. It's a firm piece of foam—there are degrees of softness, it's not like a stone—shaped like a cylinder. It's kind of like a big rolling pain that you can use to roll out the rigid knots in your body. You lie on it and the weight of your body presses into it. Then you gently roll back and forth, breaking up the tough spots with the roller.

Foam rolling can be mildly painful, but no more than a deep tissue massage. And the more often you do it, the less discomfort you'll feel.

Commitment: Buy an inexpensive foam roller and start easing into it with daily practice.

Journal...

Invest In The Right Pillow

"No one realizes how beautiful it is to travel until he comes home and rests his head on his old, familiar pillow."
– Lin Yutang

To-Do's		Long-Term Goals
✔	We spend nearly a third of our lives sleeping. That's a lot of nights, and the position your neck and head are in while you are asleep catches up to you, for better or worse.	☐
✔	Splurging on a good pillow is not a splurge at all when you take the long view. Find a pillow that supports your head and does not leave you with morning soreness. **It's an**	☐
✔	**incredible hassle to wake up, open your eyes, and immediately know that the tone of your day is set because your neck hurts right out of the gate.**	☐
✔		☐
✔	Go into a store and try a few different pillows. Find one that does not cause you any strain. Buy it from a store that will let you return it if it doesn't work out. Then, test it with a	☐
✔	couple of night's sleep. If it causes you any discomfort in the morning, or keeps you awake at night, return it and try again. There's no reason not to have the right pillow.	☐
✔		☐
✔	**Commitment:** Go get a new pillow if you have problems with your current one. Experiment until you find the one that works.	☐

Journal...

Do Not Criticize

"When we judge or criticize another person, it says nothing about that person; it merely says something about our own need to be critical." – Richard Carlson

To-Do's

- ✔
- ✔
- ✔
- ✔
- ✔
- ✔
- ✔

It's easy to criticize others. Perhaps it's a natural trait. Perhaps it's simply a learned behavior. It's an easy way to elevate ourselves--at least in our own minds, or in the eyes of people we might be showing off for. It's a convenient mask for our own insecurities. But in all my years of life, I've come to learn this one truth: **the cause of all unhappiness is criticism.** "Constructive" criticism is a lie.

Criticism leads nowhere. It's a no-win game. It produces nothing, with the possible exception of producing pain in the person we love yet are criticizing. We would never want anyone saying unnecessarily mean things about us, or judging us unfairly for sport. Why would we do the same to someone else?

Commitment: If you think you are the smartest, most observant, or detailed person, today commit to withholding every comment or remark you are tempted to make, *especially* if it's something you do for laughs. Instead, give the person a complement.

Long-Term Goals

- ☐
- ☐
- ☐
- ☐
- ☐
- ☐
- ☐

Journal...

_____
_____
_____
_____
_____
_____
_____
_____
_____
_____
_____
_____
_____
_____
_____
_____
_____
_____
_____
_____
_____
_____

Does This Really Matter?

"We learned about honesty and integrity - that the truth matters... that you don't take shortcuts or play by your own set of rules... and success doesn't count unless you earn it fair and square." – Michelle Obama

To-Do's

- ✓
- ✓
- ✓
- ✓
- ✓
- ✓
- ✓
- ✓
- ✓
- ✓
- ✓

Long-Term Goals

- ☐
- ☐
- ☐
- ☐
- ☐
- ☐
- ☐
- ☐
- ☐
- ☐
- ☐

Do you remember High School? Where the highs were insanely high, and the lows made you feel like the bottom had dropped out of the universe itself? It was a time, for so many of us, of impossible levels of melodrama. We should be able to look back at the kids we were with affection, but not necessarily emulate them in all things when it comes to perspective.

When we were children, everything felt like it mattered so much. In children this can be charming. **In adults, the tendency to treat everything as life and death is a recipe for exhaustion, stress, and burnout.** The truth is that *not everything matters,* not in the long term. Had a bad day? Will it be tormenting you a year from now? Lost a job, or a friend? Of course it matters, but will it define the years to come in an expansive way?

It is, in some ways, a sad fact that we can truly get over anything. This alone is evidence that our feelings and stresses, no matter how potent and maddening, are fleeting. They will be replaced by other challenges, other events, other days, and other memories.

Commitment: The next time you feel like the sky is falling, ask yourself how long what you are feeling in the moment will stick with you. Is it still going to matter in a month? In a year? If not, breathe, watch yourself, and try to keep perspective.

Journal...

_____
_____
_____
_____
_____
_____
_____
_____
_____
_____
_____
_____
_____
_____
_____
_____
_____
_____

Reduce The Caffeine

"Widespread caffeine use explains a lot about the twentieth century." – Greg Egan

To-Do's		Long-Term Goals
✔	Caffeine can be a wonderful aid, whether you start your day with a diet soda or you mainline espresso like so many in the working world. It can sharpen your focus, boost your energy, and help you feel like a superhero...until you crash.	☐
✔	A dependence on caffeine—you probably know what I'm talking about—is not a good thing. Any time we *need* something external to feel normal, or get through our day, or our work, we've become dependent. **The problem with caffeine dependency is that our ability to choose *not* to partake is compromised.** If you can't function without it, you're no longer as free as you could be, and it's hard to put a positive spin on that.	☐
✔		☐
✔		☐
✔		☐
✔	Excessive caffeine can also raise blood pressure, increase the likelihood of insomnia, headaches, allergies, and more.	☐
✔	**Commitment:** Reduce your caffeine intake by 50% for a week. If it's a hellacious challenge, now you know more about your dependency.	☐

Journal...

_____
_____
_____
_____
_____
_____
_____
_____
_____
_____
_____
_____
_____
_____
_____
_____
_____
_____
_____
_____
_____
_____
_____
_____

Don't Change Everything At Once

"A change in bad habits leads to a change in life." – Jenny Craig

To-Do's		Long-Term Goals

When New Years rolls around, many of us make a legion of resolutions. You might come up with so many goals that it's hard to even keep track of them all, let alone make progress on them. And each goal is generally made of smaller goals, each of which probably requires diligent, patient practice, spread out over many days.

Fitness is an easy example, and a perennial resolution. "Okay, from this point forward I'm going to exercise every day, drink eight glasses of water, lose all my fat, gain ten pounds of muscle, get cardio daily, go for a walk every afternoon, fast four times per month, do a detox juice cleanse every eight days..." Does this sound like you? Or anyone you know?

It is really, really hard to change everything at once. But small changes can pay off in big ways, and the breaking (or formation) of one habit can make it easier to change (or break) other habits. At the outset, if you have a smorgasbord of fitness goals to choose from, *just pick one and stick to it.* **We can always do one thing better.**

Commitment: Choose one habit and make a change. Give it a month. Then add another habit once the first has been formed. You won't get overwhelmed and you'll set yourself up for greater future success.

Journal...

Do An Exercise Every Time You...

"A baseball swing is a very finely tuned instrument. It is repetition, and more repetition, then a little more after that."—Reggie Jackson

To-Do's		Long-Term Goals

✔

✔

✔

✔

✔

✔

✔

✔

"If only I had time to exercise..." is a common refrain. Life can get busy in a hurry. In some ways, fitness and strength are skills. Skills require practice. **This is where you can make progress with very little effort.** You might not build a massive body or lose all of your excess weight, but you can still get so much done in very little time with a little planning.

Say that your goal was to increase your functional fitness by doing 100 squats every day. But maybe you don't have time to do a workout with 100 squats in it. Well, what if you did a few squats every time you walked by your desk? Or every 15 minutes? Surely you could free up the time for a few reps with nothing but your bodyweight?

If there is an exercise or movement you'd like to improve at, just come up with a plan and do a few reps of it every time you_____ you fill in the blank.

Commitment: Work up to 100 reps a day, with many short sequences. We all have a little extra *umph* in us.

☐
☐
☐
☐
☐
☐
☐
☐

Journal...

Forgive Someone

"Forgiveness is better than revenge; for forgiveness is the sign of a gentle nature." – Epictetus

To-Do's		Long-Term Goals

Resentment erodes your soul and well-being. And what resentments sting as badly as the wrongs which others have done to us? Harsh words, inconsiderate actions, lies, abuse...these things can linger and fester and dog us across the years.

Forgiving someone who has hurt you is easier said than done. But our time is the only truly finite resource we have. Do you really think anyone makes it to their deathbed, looks back, and says, "If only I had spent more time resenting people," or "If only I hadn't forgiven so many people..."? Of course not.

Saying, "I will forgive, but not forget," is the same as saying, "I will not forgive." When you forgive, you need to forgive AND forget. If you can do it, it's always worth it. **And of course, the hardest person to forgive can be yourself.**

Commitment: Make a list of people you would like to forgive. Choose one and figure out how to do it. Forgive, forget, and move on.

Journal...

Take Time To Laugh (Preferably With Someone You Love)

"Laughter is the shortest distance between two people." – Victor Borge

To-Do's		Long-Term Goals

It feels good to laugh, but it's an odd response to an event. Think about it. Your abdomen constricts, you start to pant. You may laugh so hard that tears roll down your face, and when it's over, you're depleted, but in the best way.

"Laughter is a form of internal jogging," Berk says in the article *The Funny Thing About Laughing (Time. 1/17/2005,)*. "What a nice way to get the lungs to move and the blood to circulate."

Consider that it may not be the laughter itself that feels so good, but the situations in which laughter is most likely to occur--gatherings with friends, families, comedies at the movie theater, and any other light-hearted circumstances.

Commitment: Watch this short video, Most Contagious Laugh, and try to breathe afterwards:

https://www.youtube.com/watch?v=mIfhOF-w1XI

Journal...

Leave Your Shoes At The Door

"I was sad because I had no shoes, until I met a man who had no feet. So I said, "Got any shoes you're not using?" – Steven Wright

To-Do's		Long-Term Goals
✔	A University of Arizona Study concluded that nine different types of bacteria clung to footwear; they can number in the millions per shoe (*Get Rid of Germs, Current Health, 2009*).	☐
✔	Would you prefer that they wait outside, or at least near your front door, or that they have free reign of your kitchen, bathroom, dining room, bedroom, etc?	☐
✔	**It's such a small change that could make a big difference in your levels of frustration with cleanliness.** Leave your	☐
✔	shoes near the entrance when you come home, and you greatly reduce the amount of germs that spread throughout	☐
✔	your home. It's a no-brainer. And you will have fewer messes to clean up if you never have anyone tracking in	☐
✔	mud, dirt, gravel, spurs, or anything else that can accumulate while walking around with shoes.	☐
✔	**Commitment:** Get a shoe rack or even a large mat where you can place your shoes when you come home, and ask your guests to do the same when they visit.	☐

Journal...

_____
_____
_____
_____
_____
_____
_____
_____
_____
_____
_____
_____
_____
_____
_____
_____
_____
_____
_____
_____
_____
_____

Prepare Food In Advance For The Week

"If you fail to plan, you are planning to fail!" – Benjamin Franklin

To-Do's		Long-Term Goals

✔

✔

✔

✔

✔

✔

✔

✔

Eating on the run requires compromises. Preparing food at home doesn't. If you know you're going to have a busy week coming up, full of intangibles and potential schedule changes, what are the chances that you will have total control over your menu and food options?

I had a friend who didn't work out on Sundays, but used them as a staging ground for the next week's strength training to come. He'd take about an hour and prepare everything he would need to make sure his nutritional needs were met. Then he was able to spend the rest of the week thinking about other things, and making the most of his training.

And many of the foods that give the most bang for their buck don't require much prep. It's not hard to put together a Tupperware dish for Monday that has a bunch of nuts, yogurt, salad, and a protein bar.

Commitment: If you have Sundays off, treat preparing some food for the week as that day's workout. Buy a few small Tupperware containers and spend a week observing how much easier this can make it to stay on track with your nutrition.

☐ ☐ ☐ ☐ ☐ ☐ ☐

Journal...

_____
_____
_____
_____
_____
_____
_____
_____
_____
_____
_____
_____
_____
_____
_____
_____
_____
_____
_____
_____
_____
_____

Learn To Enjoy Being Alone

"I owe my solitude to other people." – Alan Watts

To-Do's

✓

✓

✓

✓

✓

✓

✓

✓

✓

✓

Long-Term Goals

☐

☐

☐

☐

☐

☐

☐

☐

☐

☐

Other people can be the best, and worst, part of life. Few things are as wonderful as hanging with friends and family, having an active social life, and an endless variety of activities involving other people. Unless, of course, you're keeping yourself busy and social because you do not like your own company.

Twenty years ago, if you were alone and your friends were busy, your options for reaching out were limited. Now, picture yourself sitting in a room alone with your smartphone. You have only to send a text or post a status update on Facebook, and you will receive near-instant acknowledgement of your existence and importance to someone else.

There's nothing wrong with this, unless you really just can't handle being alone. If this is you, ask yourself where your intolerance for alone time comes from. If you are with other people, it is much harder to engage in committed introspection. **And self-reflection is necessary for real self-love.**

Commitment: Spend 30 minutes today just sitting. No phone, no texts, no computer. You don't even have to meditate if that's not your thing. Just sit and *be*. Get to know yourself again.

Journal...

Write Down The Things You Are Grateful For

"As we express our gratitude, we must never forget that the highest appreciation is not to utter words, but to live by them." – John F. Kennedy

To-Do's		Long-Term Goals

To-Do's

- ✔
- ✔
- ✔
- ✔
- ✔
- ✔
- ✔
- ✔

When life is not going well, it is easy to fixate on the negative. You can forget that there's anything good about your life, or that there ever has been.

Unless you write it down. If you can make yourself be honest and objective, there is always something positive. Making a list of the good things in your life puts it in perspective. If you take five minutes, you will think of something. If you write it down, you'll be forced to acknowledge that it is a reality.

It might not immediately make you feel better, but if you keep doing it, the list will grow. This is a way to prove to yourself that there are good things about your life, and about yourself. **No matter how down on yourself and your life you may get, there will come a point when your gratitude journal is too thick for you to ignore.**

Commitment: Get a small notebook and use it as a gratitude journal. Every day, write down at least three things that you are grateful for. Refer to it when you feel hopeless or overwhelmed.

Long-Term Goals

- ☐
- ☐
- ☐
- ☐
- ☐
- ☐
- ☐
- ☐

Journal...

_____
_____
_____
_____
_____
_____
_____
_____
_____
_____
_____
_____
_____
_____
_____
_____
_____
_____
_____
_____
_____
_____

Play "It Could Be Worse"

"To change ourselves effectively, we first had to change our perceptions." – Steven R. Covey

To-Do's

- ✔
- ✔
- ✔
- ✔
- ✔
- ✔
- ✔
- ✔
- ✔

Long-Term Goals

- ☐
- ☐
- ☐
- ☐
- ☐
- ☐
- ☐
- ☐
- ☐

This might sound a little grim, but there's a point. When we really get revved up and are trying to convince ourselves that everything is horrid, we are actually being naive and indulging in a willful act of ignorance. **We *know* that people have it worse than us. We *know* it.** Take a minute and read through a few news headlines. The chances of you reading every headline and saying "Yes, I'd totally trade my situation for the plight of this person in this horrible news story" is almost nil.

And we *know* this. But, instead of beating ourselves up and saying "Of course we're the kind of people who would make too much of our own misery," let's play a game. The game is called "It could be worse."

When you feel like you're at rock bottom, think about what would make your situation worse. There's always something. There are always a *million* things. This isn't an instant fix, but it might change the language you use to describe your situation, and your mind--and eventually your behavior--will follow suit.

Commitment: Play the game as often as you need to. Play it with a friend, who is also down on herself.

Journal...

Get A Grip

"If you keep getting stronger, there's going to come a point where you'll be able to lift more weight than you'll be able to hold onto." – Josh Hanagarne

To-Do's		Long-Term Goals
✔	They say you're only as strong as your weakest link. For many of us, even for fitness nuts, our grip strength might be the weakest link. Getting stronger hands is one of the most practical forms of strength training you can do.	☐
✔		☐
✔	It's also kind of a fun way to show off. When a giant guy swaggers in, you might think he looks strong and could probably lift a lot. **But hands, even the strongest hands in the world, still just look like hands.** It's startling to watch someone demonstrate a truly formidable grip. But no matter how powerful a grip, a strong hand is still capable of the gentlest touch.	☐
✔		☐
✔		☐
✔	There are three types of hand strength: grip, which is squeezing. Pinch grip, which is exactly what it sounds like, and support grip, which means squeezing with an open hand: think about holding a soda can and squeezing it and you'll get the idea.	☐
✔		☐
✔	**Commitment:** Buy a set of grippers, and add a couple of sets of pinch exercises to your workout routines. It's about how much pressure you can generate. For instance, grip the edge of a table or desk with your fingertips. Think about pressing them through the surface. Hold for as long as you can. You'll see your hand strength improve quickly.	☐
✔		☐
✔		☐

Journal...

Improve Your Balance

"Life is like riding a bicycle. To keep your balance, you must keep moving." – Albert Einstein

To-Do's		Long-Term Goals

✔

✔

✔

✔

✔

✔

✔

✔

✔

Have you ever felt so ungainly that you couldn't walk in a straight line while you were sober? Our feet, ankles, and knees can all go screwy and throw off our balance, as can all of the many asymmetries that develop with age and habit, not to mention those invisible cracks in the sidewalk that jump up and trip you...

Having a poor sense of balance can cause all sorts of problems, and you need not be on a balance beam to realize it. If your balance is poor, you may be dealing with inner ear and equilibrium issues. It can also mean that your ankles are weak, your feet are pointed outwards or inwards to undesirable degrees, you have inadequate posture, and more. If you can't walk a straight line smoothly, then there are problems to address.

We never want to be or feel any clumsier than we have to. We may never have perfect balance, but it can always be improved.

Commitment: Watch this short "Ask Dr. Jo" video on simple exercises to improve your balance, and implement the easy steps it demonstrates:

https://www.youtube.com/watch?v=Nc62Ju2kUAc

☐ ☐ ☐ ☐ ☐ ☐ ☐ ☐ ☐

Journal...

Ask Someone What Your Weaknesses Are

"My attitude is that if you push me towards something that you think is a weakness, then I will turn that perceived weakness into a strength." – Michael Jordan

To-Do's

- ✔
- ✔
- ✔
- ✔
- ✔
- ✔
- ✔
- ✔
- ✔
- ✔

Long-Term Goals

- ☐
- ☐
- ☐
- ☐
- ☐
- ☐
- ☐
- ☐
- ☐

Even if we say we want honest feedback on behalf of self improvement, it can be a jarring experience. Self scrutiny is admirable, but when you start turning over the rocks of your life, you do not always get to choose what is beneath them. Even more challenging is this: no one can help you understand your weaknesses better than those who have spent the most time with you, and that probably means your friends and loved ones.

No matter how committed we are to studying ourselves, another set of eyes is needed for more objectivity. If you've ever written a few pages of anything, you may have seen that you lose the ability to see your own typos. This is similar. It's hard to be as honest with ourselves as someone else can be.

But if you really want to know, you'll be motivated, not threatened, by whatever the responses are. Choose the right person, listen thoughtfully, and think about their suggestions.

Commitment: Ask someone you trust to openly and calmly discuss with you what they think your weaknesses are. Commit to being receptive, not defensive. Ask for clarification. Implement any suggestions you think would benefit you.

Journal...

_____
_____
_____
_____
_____
_____
_____
_____
_____
_____
_____
_____
_____
_____
_____
_____
_____
_____
_____

Plan Your Cheat Foods

"Pasta doesn't make you fat. How much pasta you eat makes you fat." – Giada De Laurentiis

To-Do's

- ✔
- ✔
- ✔
- ✔
- ✔
- ✔
- ✔
- ✔
- ✔
- ✔

Long-Term Goals

- ☐
- ☐
- ☐
- ☐
- ☐
- ☐
- ☐
- ☐

If you never get to indulge in your favorite foods, your chances of sticking to your nutritional plan go down. Not only is it challenging to be "good" 100% of the time, it's almost impossible.

One of the most useful traits an organism can have is adaptability. If you *never* indulge in anything outside of your normal nutritional routine, when you're eventually forced to—say you're traveling and you just have to eat a Pop Tart—it will cause you more distress than it might have if you had indulged in it sparsely.

Having a donut once a month isn't going to kill you or drastically derail your fitness goals, if you plan on it. A cheat meal shouldn't lead you into a junk food bender. It will, however, make it so you don't have to fight the cravings as often. We often want what we can't have. If we know that a reasonable portion of something "forbidden" is on the way, it can be enough to satiate that craving.

Commitment: Give yourself one "cheat window" or "cheat meal" each week so that you always know you're counting down to something that you can enjoy in that special way that only junk food seems to produce in us. Then get back to business. But over time, you will need to lessen the importance of these indulgences.

Journal...

_____
_____
_____
_____
_____
_____
_____
_____
_____
_____
_____
_____
_____
_____
_____
_____
_____
_____
_____

Volunteer, Even If You Don't Want To

"Research has shown that people who volunteer often live longer." – Allan Klein

To-Do's		Long-Term Goals

To-Do's
- ✓
- ✓
- ✓
- ✓
- ✓
- ✓
- ✓
- ✓

Time is our most finite resource. **Donating your time to a person or cause is one of the most selfless things we can do.** The easiest way to forget about yourself for a while—and this is often what is most needed when we can't feel good about ourselves—is to serve others.

Perspective is everything. If you are serving someone else, whether it's making sandwiches at a shelter, fostering pets, donating your time to a local church or youth center, you will encounter the challenges of others. Maybe your challenges are greater, maybe not, but it will provide perspective. New tools to evaluate your own situation can be found through volunteerism.

There is usually someone else suffering worse, and handling it better. Volunteering provides a way to stay humble, helpful, and to feel closer to other people who are also struggling.

Commitment: Find somewhere to volunteer for one hour this month.

Long-Term Goals
- ☐
- ☐
- ☐
- ☐
- ☐
- ☐
- ☐
- ☐

Journal...

Improve Your Posture

"I want to get old gracefully. I want to have good posture, I want to be healthy and be an example to my children." – Sting

To-Do's		Long-Term Goals

✔

✔

✔

✔

✔

✔

✔

✔

In some ways, **you *are* your spine.** It determines how good you can feel, it's full of pain sensors, it connects to your brain stem and impacts your brain function, and more. It's a good idea to keep the spine healthy, and one of the easiest ways to do this is simply to improve your posture.

Over time, your spine can settle into positions that can lead to pinched nerves, chronic pain, and more. Picture a person sitting at a computer. The head is probably sitting far forward on the neck, the shoulders are probably hunched forward, etc. Think about the position of the spine. This seated position could not look less natural!

Back pain is such a distraction, and it can creep into everything we do. Taking time each day to gradually put your head, neck, and spine back into optimal position will pay off for your entire life.

Commitment: Read *The Egoscue Method of Health Through Motion.* It's a simple introduction to balancing body asymmetries and improving posture.

http://www.amazon.com/Egoscue-Method-Health-Through-Motion/dp/0060924306/ref=sr_1_1?ie=UTF8&qid=1455727990&sr=8-1&keywords=the+egoscue+method

Long-Term Goals checkboxes: ☐ ☐ ☐ ☐ ☐ ☐ ☐ ☐

Journal...

_____
_____
_____
_____
_____
_____
_____
_____
_____
_____
_____
_____
_____
_____
_____
_____
_____
_____
_____
_____
_____

Use Sunscreen

"I can only be in the sun for 15 minutes before burning. I have sunscreen on my face every day. If I'm walking on the sunny side of the street, I'll walk to the shady side. I'm too uncomfortable in the sun." – Julianne Moore

To-Do's

- ✔
- ✔
- ✔
- ✔
- ✔
- ✔
- ✔
- ✔

You might have fond memories of childhood in which you ran around all day with no sunscreen, happy as a lark. You may also have fears of being older and paying the price for those sunshiny days. The truth is, sunshine is still a good source of Vitamin D, and going outside is still a good thing. But the days of consequence-free days in the sun are gone. Just Google "the ozone layer," and you will quickly learn why we should be afraid.

Sunscreen is the antidote. If you put sunscreen on before spending significant time outdoors, you can still reap the benefits of sunlight without the damage that its harsh rays can cause you. There are sprays and creams for every skin type and shade. It's gotten to the point where there's just no excuse for not putting on sunscreen, and it only takes a couple of minutes. **Your skin is your largest organ, after all.**

Commitment: Use sunscreen when you spend more than thirty minutes outside. Get a high SPF and enjoy your skin for the rest of your life.

Long-Term Goals

- ☐
- ☐
- ☐
- ☐
- ☐
- ☐
- ☐
- ☐

Journal...

February 27

Take Vitamins

"To all my little Hulkamaniacs, say your prayers, take your vitamins and you will never go wrong." – Hulk Hogan

To-Do's
✔
✔
✔
✔
✔
✔
✔
✔
✔

Long-Term Goals
☐ ☐ ☐ ☐ ☐ ☐ ☐ ☐ ☐

No matter how healthy your eating habits are, there is still a chance that you could be nutritionally deficient in some areas. Eating nothing but salad might make you lean and mean, with the body fat of a statue, but you probably won't be getting any vitamin B12. If you cut out dairy you might experience less congestion and avoid the chemicals of modern day dairy production, but you might not get enough calcium without a plan.

A good multivitamin can help you cover your bases. It also takes a lot of the guesswork out of things. No matter how meticulously you're willing to be when planning meals, do you really want to say, "Hmm, did I get enough Manganese, Selenium, Pantothenic Acid, Biotin, Chromium," and on an on ad nauseum? Probably not.

But if you're willing to get in the habit of swallowing a couple of pills with breakfast, you'll be set.

Commitment: Get a good multivitamin and take it daily. If you lift weights, consider Animal Pak. It's the most comprehensive multivitamin for people who put serious demands on their bodies through exercise.

Journal...

Eat Breakfast

"What nicer thing can you do for somebody than make them breakfast?" – Anthony Bourdain

To-Do's		Long-Term Goals
✔	Making breakfast for *yourself* is also one of the nicest things you can do for someone, namely, you. Nearly every cereal commercial you've ever seen tells you that breakfast is the most important meal of the day. It's not just a marketing sound byte. Food is *fuel.* For your brain, body, and performance, whether that means going for a run or just going to work with an alert, sharp mind.	☐
✔		☐
✔		☐
✔	And when do you most feel like you need fuel? After a night of sleep, during which, you aren't feeding your body. When do you need to be most alert and have the greatest powers of concentration? Probably when you go to work. Food also gets your metabolism going for the day. It's best to start that engine revving early.	☐
✔		☐
✔		☐
✔	The other side of breakfast is to **make sure it's a *good* breakfast.** Back to the sound byte--you want a balanced breakfast. Get some protein, good fats, and carbs. A green smoothie can be a great choice. I have one most mornings. You will feel better, think better, be more productive physically, and look forward to your day more. Dragging yourself through a shift at work can be a bummer. Give yourself a chance to feel as good as you can, as soon into the day as you can.	☐
✔		☐
✔		☐
✔	**Commitment:** Simple. Eat a balanced breakfast every day. If you're not doing this, start tomorrow morning. Download my book, "Healthy Green Smoothies: 50 Easy Recipes That Will Change Your Life."	☐

Journal...

_____
_____
_____
_____
_____
_____
_____
_____
_____
_____
_____
_____
_____
_____
_____
_____
_____

Celebrate The Unexpected

"The marvels of daily life are exciting; no movie director can arrange the unexpected that you find in the street."
– Robert Doisneau

To-Do's		Long-Term Goals

Just in case you're reading this on a Leap Year, this tip is a reminder that oddities abound in all walks of life. **Usually, when someone says "I'm bored," they're just not paying attention.** There is always something to learn, something strange, something unexpected happening just beyond the edges of your vision.

The random chaos and craziness of simply being alive virtually *ensures* that boredom can be vanquished, provided you're not in the middle of some tedious task that is dull and repetitive by definition.

But the world is a whimsical, unpredictable, and kooky place. And as long as it's filled with wonderful, fallible, emotional people, that's never going to change.

Commitment: The next time you feel the tedium of routine, make an extra effort to look around and find something surprising. Start with something that has unexpectedly happened in your life. Then write it down in your gratitude journal.

Journal...

March

Practice Empathy

"The struggle of my life created empathy - I could relate to pain, being abandoned, having people not love me."
– Oprah Winfrey

To-Do's		Long-Term Goals
✔	Empathy is the ability to understand what another person is feeling and thinking, and to see yourself in their position. Why would you want to do this? Because you're *part of a human condition.* Unless you're a sociopath, you are connected to other people emotionally, for better or worse. **One of the best ways to ease your own suffering is to try to make someone else's situation easier.**	☐
✔		☐
✔		☐
✔	You can only help someone as well as you can understand them. The feeling of empathy is natural, but the practice of it, less so. True empathy requires you to slow down and genuinely try to understand and feel what someone is going through. It requires you to try to comprehend, not how you would feel in their situation, but how *they* are actually feeling, based on what you know about them.	☐
✔		☐
✔		☐
✔	It requires asking, patience, compassion, and a willingness to set aside judgment. You must sit quietly and listen intently. There is no downside to empathy, and it will give you the ability to help others when they can't help themselves feel better.	☐
✔		☐
✔	**Commitment:** Listen to a person today, who is struggling. It can be a friend, family, or stranger. Try to understand their situation through their eyes, not yours.	☐

Journal...

_____
_____
_____
_____
_____
_____
_____
_____
_____
_____
_____
_____
_____
_____
_____
_____
_____
_____
_____
_____

Clean Pain vs. Dirty Pain

"Pain can be the best teacher you'll ever have, if it changes your behavior." – Adam T. Glass

To-Do's

✔

✔

✔

✔

✔

✔

✔

✔

✔

✔

Long-Term Goals

☐

☐

☐

☐

☐

☐

☐

☐

☐

☐

Pain is a part of life. Sometimes things--body, mind, emotions--are just going to hurt. But there are important distinctions to be made between pain and suffering, and of the different types of emotional pain. Dr. Steven Hayes, noted psychologist, gives what is perhaps the clearest and most useful distinction between what he calls "clean pain" and "dirty pain."

Clean pain is natural. It is the sprained ankle. The scraped knee. The bumped head. The discomfort the day after the slip on the ice. Clean pain does not come with an elaborate story attached to it. "I sprained my ankle. The End."

Dirty pain spins the stories into something personal and inward-directed. "Only someone as stupid as *me* would sprain their ankle." "Of *course* I slipped on the ice, I'm a clumsy oaf." **Dirty pain is a chance to torment ourselves for natural events** that do not deserve to be blown out of proportion. And no matter how trivial the dirty pain, it still leaves a scar.

Commitment: The next time something hurts, breathe calmly and think. Ask yourself if you are experiencing clean or dirty pain. If you decide that the pain is unnatural, or dirty, change the story you are telling yourself. Or, if you can't do that, just recognize that you are beating yourself up, and try to determine the reason why.

Journal...

_____
_____
_____
_____
_____
_____
_____
_____
_____
_____
_____
_____
_____
_____
_____
_____
_____
_____
_____

Pain Isn't Necessarily A Symptom

"Life is difficult. This is a great truth, one of the greatest truths. It is a great truth because once we truly see this truth, we transcend it. Once we truly know that life is difficult—once we truly understand and accept it—then life is no longer difficult. Because once it is accepted, the fact that life is difficult no longer matters." – M. Scott Peck

To-Do's		Long-Term Goals
✔	There's nothing wrong with saying that life can be unfair. At times, it is a downright brutal (and painful) business. Sometimes being realistic can look like pessimism. But describing a negative situation realistically is not pessimistic. It can be healthy because it is honest. Trouble sets in when the *only* thing you find yourself saying is, "It's not fair! It hurts! It's too hard! It wasn't supposed to be like this!"	☐
✔		☐
✔		☐
✔	Wishing things had gone another way is the height of futility. Every day you have lived is now past. It *did not* go another way. All you truly have to work with is what you do today, and what you do next. This can be a painful realization at first. But it's always healthier to be honest about what's happening. Life is hard. Sometimes it will hurt. And that's fine. **You'll always get to the other side of it.** To date, you have survived every "this is the hardest day of my life" day.	☐
✔		☐
✔		☐
✔	**Commitment:** The next time you are hurting, tell yourself that it's okay. You're not doing anything wrong just because you're in pain. Pay attention to it. Note the physical and emotional reactions you're having. Breathe. It will pass.	☐
✔		☐

Journal...

_____
_____
_____
_____
_____
_____
_____
_____
_____
_____
_____
_____
_____
_____
_____
_____
_____
_____

Keep Promises To Yourself

"A promise made is a debt unpaid." – Robert W. Service

To-Do's		Long-Term Goals

Most of us would never break a promise to a friend or loved one. No one wants to be a liar, or to be seen as a liar by others. But if you've ever had the experience of seeing yet another one of your New Year's Resolutions go the way of the dodo, you know that **lying to yourself is much easier.**

When you tell yourself that you're going to lose weight, workout more, read more, write more, spend more time with friends, drink less, and then you stop working on it, or you never even start, then you've broken a promise to yourself. It's easier because nobody knows about the lie except you. And it's not like you're hurting anyone else, right?

Wrong. One of the greatest gifts you can give yourself is to treat the promises you make to yourself as seriously as the promises you make to others.

Commitment: Did you make a resolution this year? If you did, and you have let it slide, recommit to it today. Take the first small step back to it as soon as possible. Be gentle with yourself when you misstep, but ask yourself why you don't treat promises to yourself as seriously as those you make to others.

Journal...

Learn To Say No

"The art of pleasing is the art of deception." – Luc de Clapiers

To-Do's		**Long-Term Goals**

✓

✓

✓

✓

✓

✓

✓

✓

✓

How well do you protect yourself from others? That question isn't meant to sound overly dramatic, as if you're a castle under siege from invading friends, family members, and co-workers. Let's rephrase: do you have time that you guard fiercely for yourself? Time to do whatever helps you recharge?

The people most likely to set inadequate boundaries with others are the people pleasers. There's nothing wrong with wanting to make other people happy, or to be useful, or help whoever you can help, *as long as* you don't neglect yourself in the process. If you're rushing around helping other people so much that your own needs go unmet, it's not healthy.

In order to be able to say no when you need to, **you need to know what you want for yourself**, so this is a tandem goal. Think about what your passion is, and the goals you want to achieve, and then decide to carve out time for them/you.

Commitment: Choose a goal. Decide what needs to happen in order for you to work on it daily. Then commit to saying no as much as you need to in order to accomplish the day task.

Journal...

Know Your Identity Outside Of Your Relationships

"Know thyself." – Delphic Maxim, often attributed to Socrates

To-Do's		Long-Term Goals

Who are you? What would you like people to know about you? How would you like them to describe you? What do you value most in yourself?

Some people do not have any sense of identity, other than what they mean to another person. If all of your self-worth comes from another person's validation, whether it's a father, mother, sibling, or lover, **what are you going to do during the times when you may have none of those?**

You are one entire person, full of your own memories, experiences, and unique potential. You are not half of a whole.

Commitment: Love yourself, and then you can learn to love others better. Be honest, and think about whether you feel that you have worth on your own, or if it comes from external sources. Watch this brief TED Talk by Hetain Patel, Who Am I?

https://www.youtube.com/watch?v=FPhHHtn8On8

To-Do's checkmarks: ✔ ✔ ✔ ✔ ✔ ✔ ✔ ✔

Long-Term Goals checkboxes: ☐ ☐ ☐ ☐ ☐ ☐ ☐ ☐

Journal...

Don't Apologize More Than Is Necessary

"More people should apologize, and more people should accept apologies when sincerely made." – Greg Lemond

To-Do's		Long-Term Goals

Pay attention to the way people speak on any given day and you'll hear a staggering amount of apologies. "Sorry sorry sorry." Someone might apologize to you for nearly bumping into you, for staring a second too long, for nothing at all, it seems. And then, of course, the people who truly wrong us never seem to be in a hurry to say sorry.

This isn't just semantics. **You can tell a lot about someone by the language they use.** Someone who apologizes constantly, even if it's well-intentioned or looks like politeness, has an apologetic mindset. Part of them is assuming that they are fault for more things than they should be taking upon themselves.

If you're always apologizing, ask yourself why. Ask yourself if you are really messing up as often as you seem to think you are.

Commitment: Only apologize when an apology is truly necessary. And when people apologize to you, accept their apologies quickly and graciously.

Journal...

Find The "Right Way" To Exercise For You

"To enjoy the glow of good health, you must exercise." – Gene Tunney, Boxing Champion

To-Do's

- ✔
- ✔
- ✔
- ✔
- ✔
- ✔
- ✔
- ✔
- ✔
- ✔
- ✔
- ✔

Long-Term Goals

- ☐
- ☐
- ☐
- ☐
- ☐
- ☐
- ☐
- ☐
- ☐
- ☐
- ☐
- ☐

We all know we should exercise. We're all told constantly about the benefits, and hopefully there are times when you've experienced all of the gifts that exercise can give, even if you're not currently in the habit. And that's the key word here: *habit.*

Unfortunately, developing the exercise habit in no way guarantees that exercise is suddenly fun or enjoyable for you. The key to longevity in exercise is to find a type of exercise that you enjoy. If you enjoy it, you can look forward to it. If you look forward to it, it's self-obvious: you'll keep doing it, and making time for it. It's so obvious that it shouldn't even need to be said: **We like to do what we like to do.**

The problem is that "exercise" and "fitness" are narrow terms. They conjure up exercise routines and templates, which can give you the idea that there's a "right" way to exercise. *If I'm not doing what the magazine says to do, I must be making a mistake.* But exercise can be anything you want! Don't feel like you have to lift weights, or run, or swing a kettlebell, or do Crossfit, or anything that you don't enjoy, in order to "exercise." Find something fun that gets your heart rate up, keeps you moving, and that you enjoy.

Keep trying. Play racquetball. Hike. Dance. Get onto a dodgeball team. Golfing at least requires a lot of walking. Snowboard. Take a tumbling class. For me, it's hardcore gardening. Keep going until you find your sweet spot. Once you do, you'll be chomping at the bit to get back to it. There's no "right" way. There's only right for you.

Commitment: Find a physical activity that you enjoy. Practice it consistently for a month. Chances are, you'll turn that month into two.

Journal...

_____
_____
_____
_____
_____
_____
_____
_____
_____
_____
_____

Find An Open Space

"I grew up in New Mexico, and the older I get, I have less need for contemporary culture and big cities and all the stuff we are bombarded with. I am happier at my ranch in the middle of nowhere watching a bug carry leaves across the grass, listening to silence, riding my horse, and being in open space." – Tom Ford

To-Do's		Long-Term Goals
✔	Maybe you can't drop everything and go live in a ranch in the middle of nowhere like Tom Ford, but ask yourself this question: When was the last time I was out in a truly open space? If you live in a city, days, weeks, months, and even years can pass without laying eyes on an open sky, or seeing the expanse of the horizon.	☐
✔		☐
✔	**The mind and emotions experience their own forms of claustrophobia.** Even if you're a die-hard city slicker, few will dispute that there is less peace to be had in a city than in a forest or field. And again, standing in a forest or field is not essential to a happy life. But *variety* is. Periodic tranquility is never a bad thing.	☐
✔		☐
✔		☐
✔	And few things impose stillness upon us like nature. A spot to watch, breathe, and think. If nothing else, it is *different.*	☐
✔	**Commitment:** Do what it takes to get to an open space this month. Try to find a location where you can't even see a building. Make note of how you feel. Walk. Breathe. If you enjoy it, revisit this place as often as you feel the need.	☐
✔		☐

Journal...

_____
_____
_____
_____
_____
_____
_____
_____
_____
_____
_____
_____
_____
_____
_____
_____
_____
_____
_____
_____
_____

Use An Air Purifier

"There's so much pollution in the air now that if it weren't for our lungs there'd be no place to put it all." –
Robert Orben, American Comedian

To-Do's		Long-Term Goals

There's no way to stop breathing. Well, there are actually many ways, but they all lead to the same outcome. But if you want to live, you have to keep breathing, and the quality of your life can be heavily shaped by the quality of the air you breathe. Unfortunately, you can't go outside and put lids on the smokestacks, close down the foundries, get everyone to stop driving, and knock the cigarettes out of people's mouths. So you're left with the air in your home, which you have more control over.

Enter the air purifier, a simple machine that can help reduce the contaminants in the air of your home. Honestly, if you have a shot at breathing cleaner air--and you do--there's no reason not to try it.

You're going to spend every minute of your life dependent on the air you're taking in. Control what you can control.

Commitment: Buy an air purifier and see if your lungs feel better. It's an inexpensive experiment and can greatly help over the long term.

Journal...

Get A Brita

"By polluting clear water with slime you will never find good drinking water." — *Aeschylus*

To-Do's		Long-Term Goals
✔	In 2012, according to *Business Insider,* "At an average cost of $1.22 per gallon, consumers are spending 300 times the cost of tap water to drink bottled water."	☐
✔	That was four years ago, and Americans spent nearly 12 billion dollars on bottled water.	☐
✔	Not that there's anything wrong with drinking healthy water. **We're all made of the stuff**, as I'm sure you remember from elementary school. But there is a cheaper way that is just as good. Buy a water filter. You might have to refill it every couple of days, but it's not going to cost you more than the price of the pitcher--less than $30--and replacement filters--approximately $30.	☐
✔		☐
✔		☐
✔	Also keep in mind that all of that bottled water comes in plastic, and the one-use bottles wind up in landfills or in the middle of the ocean as part of a plastic conglomerate the size of Texas.	☐
✔		☐
✔	**Commitment:** Buy a Brita – or another water filter (I use ZeroWater Filter) – and let the bottles go.	☐

Journal...

_____
_____
_____
_____
_____
_____
_____
_____
_____
_____
_____
_____
_____
_____
_____
_____
_____
_____
_____
_____
_____
_____

Get A Massage

"I love a good massage, and they gotta go deep." – Zoe Lister-Jones

To-Do's		Long-Term Goals

✔

✔

✔

✔

✔

✔

✔

✔

✔

✔

If you've ever had a great massage, you've probably groaned, literally, with pleasure and relief as the fingers-- or elbows, or palms, or even knees or feet in some cases-- sink into the deep tissue that we could never reach on our own. **Suddenly it feels like *all* of our discomfort was buried in there.**

A good massage breaks up rigid tissue, loosens up tendons, releases toxins (and increases oxytocin, the hormone known sometimes as the "love hormone," and gives the body a chance to move again with better biomechanics, now that it is more relaxed and reset.

A massage from a licensed masseuse doesn't have to be costly to be effective, and you don't have to get one every week to reap the benefits, even though I do. As with many of the tips in this book, it's not really splurging on something if it actually makes you healthier and happier.

Commitment: Get a massage at least once a month from a licensed masseuse. You're probably already spending $60 a month on something that doesn't contribute to your health. Use that money to treat yourself to a good massage. To keep my body performing at a top level for surgery, I get a weekly massage.

Journal...

Consider Therapy

"Words of comfort, skillfully administered, are the oldest therapy known to man." – Louis Nizer

To-Do's		Long-Term Goals

No matter how committed you are to letting go of resentment, forgiving others, loving yourself, learning to set boundaries between you and other people, and so on, you might not be able to resolve all of your challenges on your own. **Life is a messy business, and we don't always have access to the emotions that we most need to deal with.**

A professional can help. Therapists—whether you choose a psychologist or a psychotherapist—can see you in a way that you can't, and they are trained to be objective. A good therapist will not let you off the hook for your mistakes, but will also help you see those times when you are being too hard on yourself.

Therapy has an unfortunate stereotype. It's for the weak and the whiny, or a therapist is nothing but an expensive friend. It's for people who aren't "tough" enough to face reality and "get over" their issues. None of this is true. The real value of a therapist has to be experienced to be understood.

Commitment: If you feel like you need emotional support, make an appointment with a therapist. Commit to two sessions of completely open and honest self-reflection with the guidance of a professional.

Journal...

_____
_____
_____
_____
_____
_____
_____
_____
_____
_____
_____
_____
_____
_____
_____
_____
_____
_____
_____

Replacing "But" With "And"

"Where There Is Confusion, Look First To The Language." – Christopher Hitchens

To-Do's		Long-Term Goals

✔

✔

✔

✔

✔

✔

✔

✔

Avoiding anything with the slightest negative connotation can work against us. There are challenges we need to meet head on, and pretending things are wonderful when they aren't can cause unnecessary psychological trauma.

But there are small habits we can develop that can start weeding out small forms of negativity without needing a lot of thought and planning. One of the easiest changes you can make is to replace the word "but" with the word "and."

For instance, consider the sentence, "I really want to get this job but I don't know if I'm qualified for it." What if you changed it to "I really want to get this job *and* I don't know if I'm qualified for it." **It's a small change, but one sounds more hopeful.** Changing "but" to "and" can even require you to restructure your sentences so they don't sound awkward. It would probably be more likely, in the above example, to saying something like, "I really want to get this job *and* I hope I'm qualified for it." Over time, this will help you feel more positive.

Commitment: Take one day and change *but* to *and*. If it's easy, you're on the right path. If it's hard, you could probably use permanent extension of the exercise.

☐ ☐ ☐ ☐ ☐ ☐ ☐ ☐ ☐

Journal...

_____
_____
_____
_____
_____
_____
_____
_____
_____
_____
_____
_____
_____
_____
_____
_____
_____
_____
_____
_____
_____

Tell The Truth

"Honesty is the first chapter in the book of wisdom." – Thomas Jefferson

To-Do's	
✔	
✔	
✔	
✔	
✔	
✔	
✔	
✔	

Long-Term Goals

☐
☐
☐
☐
☐
☐
☐
☐

Being lied to is a humiliating experience, even if you are unaware that it is happening. The person being lied to is acting on incomplete information, or inaccurate representations, and the liar knows that this is false, but gets to watch the other person act unaware.

If you're the one telling the lie you humiliate the other person and you erode your own integrity. We're not talking about the little white lies that we tell to spare other people's feelings. We're talking about lies that we tell to hide truths that we do not want other people to know. Lies told for gain. Lies hurt, if not the oblivious people we lie to, ourselves.

There are so few times when telling the truth is not the right choice. You can get used to lying, sadly. We can get used to anything if we do it enough. **But the more lies you tell, the more you'll form a truth for yourself that is inaccurate.** You might lose your sense of identity entirely.

Commitment: Be honest in all of your dealings with other people, especially with yourself.

Journal...

You Don't Have To Have The Last Word

"The aim of argument, or of discussion, should not be victory, but progress." – Joseph Joubert

To-Do's		Long-Term Goals

We can safely assume that most of us have been in a position where we want to have the last word. Unfortunately, this usually occurs in situations where the other person also wants to have the final say. To get in one last jab. **And behind all of the sparring is this: *I want to be right.***

True argument leads somewhere useful. It is an exchange of ideas, even if there is a combative element. Much of what is considered debate, particularly in politics, is simply very loud talking. And also, true debate is often not what is at stake when we're having arguments that feel silly to us, even as they are unfolding.

Think of a past argument you had, where you wanted the last word. Would your life have been damaged in any way if you had simply let the other person be right? If you had let them have the last word?

Commitment: If you're a person who always wants the last word, just let the other person have it the next time the opportunity arises. Sit with the agitation afterwards and ask yourself what it means, and what is truly at stake.

Journal...

Consider Acupuncture

"I'm afraid of needles, except acupuncture needles." – Catherine O'Hara

To-Do's

- ✓
- ✓
- ✓
- ✓
- ✓
- ✓
- ✓
- ✓
- ✓

Long-Term Goals

- ☐
- ☐
- ☐
- ☐
- ☐
- ☐
- ☐
- ☐
- ☐

What does the word Acupuncture make you think of? You might be picturing a scene straight out of a horror movie. Someone lying on their back, myriad needles sticking out of their forehead, arms, legs, cheeks, and way on down the line. And you might be right in asking, *Why in the world would someone do that?*

They're probably doing it because nothing else has worked for them. In *Acupuncture: History From The Yellow Emperor to Modern Anesthesia Practice,* Amanda Faircloth cites evidence for acupuncture's efficacy both as a pain reliever, and also as an anxiety reducer. It's interesting that she specifically cites its use to reduce anxiety in the minutes before someone undergoes surgery.

When it comes to wellness, we should all be results-oriented. **You want as many tools to try as possible.** Acupuncture is accessible and inexpensive, and some people say nothing else will alleviate their pain.

Commitment: Talk with a licensed acupuncturist. Consider giving it a try. Do it for fun if you're skeptical. At worst, you'll leave with a story to tell. At best, you may find something that improves your quality of life.

Journal...

_____
_____
_____
_____
_____
_____
_____
_____
_____
_____
_____
_____
_____
_____
_____
_____
_____
_____
_____
_____
_____

Keep Expanding The Toolbox

"If you try anything—if you try to lose weight, or to improve yourself, or to love, or to make the world a better place—you have already achieved something wonderful, before you even begin. Forget failure. If things don't work out the way you want, hold your head up high and be proud. And try again. And again. And again!" – Sara Dessun

To-Do's		Long-Term Goals
✔	If you deal with any sort of chronic issue—whether it's depression, fibromyalgia, insomnia, etc.—there will hopefully be times when you find something that works. Maybe it's a medication, or meditation, or a change in your diet. When you deal with long-term distress, and then something works, or seems to, it can be really tempting to get on the rooftop and scream "I've found THE answer!"	☐
✔		☐
✔		☐
✔	Resist the temptation to believe that you have found *The Answer*. Every time something good happens or a solution presents itself, reframe it as having found *an* answer. Maybe it works forever, maybe not. But during those unfortunate instances when a solution stops working, it is far less painful to know that *an* answer is no longer what it once was, versus having to let go of the idea that *The Answer* is gone forever.	☐
✔		☐
✔		☐
✔	**Not every problem has one solution.** When something is working, keep studying, keep trying new things, and gives yourself options so that you'll know what you're going to try next, if you need a change of direction.	☐
✔		☐
✔	**Commitment:** If you are dealing with a specific condition, continue studying it even during periods of relief. Once we think we know something, we often stop trying to understand it.	☐
✔		☐

Journal...

_____
_____
_____
_____
_____
_____
_____
_____
_____
_____
_____
_____
_____
_____
_____
_____

Never Stop Learning

"Live as if you were to die tomorrow. Learn as if you were to live forever." – Mahatma Gandhi

To-Do's

- ✔
- ✔
- ✔
- ✔
- ✔
- ✔
- ✔

Is there a worse lesson to teach a child than "Curiosity killed the cat?" Are you kidding me? We only have so many days to live, and to learn. **The key to constant and long-term self-improvement, above all others, is curiosity.**

Curiosity prompts us to ask questions. "What if I….?" "I wonder how that works?" Questions are the bedrock of all progress, because they lead to answers. Answers usually lead to more questions. I can't imagine someone on their deathbed exclaiming, "If only I'd learned less!"

Make this your mantra: *There is a never a reason for boredom.* You will never know everything. So you can learn every day of your life. If you never stop learning, you will always have something new to ask, and that will mean there will always be another answer to find.

Commitment: Learn something new every day. Write it down in your journal or cell phone to lock it in.

Long-Term Goals

- ☐
- ☐
- ☐
- ☐
- ☐
- ☐
- ☐

Journal...

Ask How You Would Parent Yourself

"I got a lot of support from my parents. That's the one thing I always appreciated. They didn't tell me I was being stupid; they told me I was being funny." — Jim Carrey

To-Do's
✔
✔
✔
✔
✔
✔
✔
✔
✔

We are all the products of our childhoods. There's no getting around it. If you were raised by your parents, as most people are, you are largely a product of how they parented you. If you change course later in life, or if your parents reared you in a way that requires great changes from you later in life, it can be painful.

It can be helpful, particularly if you feel resentment for your parents, to ask yourself, *Right now, if I was one of my parents, how would I parent me*? **In order to resent your parents, you must have ideas about things you wish that they had done differently.** This is a simple exercise that might give you a new perspective.

If you can't figure out exactly what you need, ask yourself what a good parent might think you need at this moment. Then, if possible, give it to yourself.

Commitment: The next time you wish things were different, put yourself in the role of your parent. Try to give yourself the same advice a kind, nurturing, insightful, dedicated parent would give. Then, have the courage to take the advice.

Long-Term Goals
☐
☐
☐
☐
☐
☐
☐
☐

Journal...

Give Up On Perfection

"Art is never finished, only abandoned." – Leonardo Da Vinci

To-Do's		Long-Term Goals

To-Do's
- ✓
- ✓
- ✓
- ✓
- ✓
- ✓
- ✓
- ✓

Long-Term Goals
- ☐
- ☐
- ☐
- ☐
- ☐
- ☐
- ☐
- ☐

It can be a hard thing to realize that there will always be someone smarter, taller, thinner, younger, wealthier, more muscular, and on and on and on. None of that means you aren't a wonderful, worthwhile human being, but there will nearly always be someone else who can do, or *is,* just a little more of that one thing that's so important to you.

We are all works of art. We can never bring ourselves to completion or perfection. So what can we shoot for instead?

Simple. **Improvement.** Every situation, every body, every book, every endeavor, every project, can be improved. You've probably heard the cliché that it's the journey, not the destination. Nowhere is this truer than of the constant ability to strive for improvement. If you think perfection is attainable, you will always be unsatisfied to some degree.

Commitment: Strive for constant improvement in the things that matter to you. Do not pretend that perfection is a reality. Just be better today than you were yesterday.

Journal...

_____
_____
_____
_____
_____
_____
_____
_____
_____
_____
_____
_____
_____
_____
_____
_____
_____
_____
_____
_____
_____
_____

Finish What You Start

"We all have dreams. But in order to make dreams come into reality, it takes an awful lot of determination, dedication, self-discipline, and effort." – Jesse Owens

To-Do's		Long-Term Goals

There are many studies suggesting that everyone thinks they have a book in them. Meaning, everyone thinks they could write a book. While it's true that everyone can start a book, the number of people who finish the writing they start is illuminating.

But we don't need to talk about writing to illustrate the principle. Think of what it feels like to need to sneeze. Now think of the relief that you feel when the sneeze is out. It resolves a very particular sort of stress. Now, think of your goals. **When you start working on them, and then abandon your projects, think of it as the sneeze that you stifled, instead of letting it out and feeling better.**

The accumulation of these unresolved stresses take a toll. What if you had held every sneeze you ever needed to let out?

Commitment: If you're in the middle of a project, especially if it's something you have a habit of abandoning or leaving undone, finish it today.

Journal...

Avoid Procrastination

"Procrastination makes easy things hard, hard things harder." – Mason Cooley

To-Do's	
✔	
✔	
✔	
✔	
✔	
✔	
✔	
✔	
✔	

Long-Term Goals

☐ ☐ ☐ ☐ ☐ ☐ ☐ ☐ ☐

Every hour ends. So does every day, year, decade, and century. Time marches on, regardless of what we want, intend, complain about, or embrace. Here's the point: If you want to accomplish something, or take a step towards a goal, today can be a day in which you took the step. The day will end either way.

If you want to exercise every day, today is a day in which you could have exercised. The day ends either way. We often put things off in favor of doing something more enjoyable in the moment, but it is also natural to avoid hard or painful tasks, even if they are critical. **Much of living in the moment involves facing head on the pain of certain moments.**

The more tasks pile up, the more cluttered your mind will be, and the more agitated your emotions. The longer you put off the things that would make you happy, the less time you have to work on them. The more time you spend doing the wrong things--wrong for *you*--the less time you have to do them right.

Commitment: Choose a task that you have been putting off. Then do it and get it behind you.

Journal...

_____
_____
_____
_____
_____
_____
_____
_____
_____
_____
_____
_____
_____
_____
_____
_____
_____
_____
_____

Forgot About The Number On The Scale

"I'm prouder of my weight loss than my Oscar!" – Jennifer Hudson

To-Do's		Long-Term Goals

The quest for more muscle and/or less body fat has granted the number on our bathroom scales an authority it does not deserve. Forget what you think you know about the magic number at which you would look "good" or "right" or "perfect."

Men often hit the number they've been chasing with countless weightlifting sessions and binge eating, only to realize that they don't look like the muscleman on the magazine cover.

Women might lose twenty pounds, hit their target weight, and realize that they still look softer or more overweight than they had expected. There are so many factors that play into body composition, **and the number on the scale might be the *least relevant.***

Commitment: Even if you're already in a committed fitness regimen, take a couple of weeks to stop weighing yourself, whether you're trying to gain or lose. Go by the mirror and see if you can observe changes that make you happy.

Journal...

Don't Work Too Much

"Choose a job you love, and you will never have to work a day in your life." – Confucius

To-Do's

- ✔
- ✔
- ✔
- ✔
- ✔
- ✔
- ✔
- ✔
- ✔

Long-Term Goals

- ☐
- ☐
- ☐
- ☐
- ☐
- ☐
- ☐
- ☐
- ☐

Being an adult can be a drag, and the fact that we need to sell our labor, skills, ideas, and time to pay for the things we need in order to survive can be a good example of this—if we're in the wrong job, or if we're in a job that requires so much from us that we can't enjoy our lives.

Unless you are independently wealthy or on unemployment, you probably have a job. If you work full-time, chances are that you spend more time with your co-workers than with your friends and family. If you don't enjoy your job, or if you spend too much time and energy on it to live in the moment frequently, it is time to ask yourself what the cost of this is.

Picture yourself on your deathbed. Imagine who is there with you. Do you wish you had given them, or yourself, more of your time? Or do you say, "Wow, I wish I'd spent more time at the office?"

Commitment: Take time for yourself and make sure you are progressing on your goals and self-fulfillment. If you hate your job, find a way to make it better or find a new one. Life is short.

Journal...

_____
_____
_____
_____
_____
_____
_____
_____
_____
_____
_____
_____
_____
_____
_____
_____
_____
_____
_____
_____
_____

Avoid Stress Eating

"To eat well in England you should have breakfast three times a day." – Somerset Maugham

To-Do's		Long-Term Goals
✔		☐
✔		☐
✔		☐
✔		☐
✔		☐
✔		☐
✔		☐
✔		☐
✔		☐
✔		☐
✔		☐
✔		☐
✔		☐

All addictions come from a similar place: an unwillingness to be uncomfortable. Now, this is a slightly reductive simplification, but the theory is sound. Our addictions provide more pleasure to us than makes sense.

With regards to stress eating, think of it as a habit, not an addiction. If you are like most people, you deal with a fair amount of anxiety. Work, family, finances, health, aging...**there are so many stresses that are simply the cost of being alive.** To feel better, some of us turn to alcohol, some to sex, some to drugs. Others turn to food. It's not hard to understand why. Food that tastes good makes you feel happy. When you want to feel happy, food is there. The anxiety goes away, or is at least mitigated by the pleasure of eating, but it comes with a toll.

Weight gain, excess body fat, an increasingly sedentary lifestyle due to diminished mobility, gastric problems, etc. These can all result from eating more often than we need to, and stress/comfort eating is, by definition, *not* eating for nutrition and fuel. It is a coping mechanism. There is always going to be stress, as long as you are alive. If you always try to eat stress in the form of food, you'll pay a price.

Commitment: Observe yourself over the next week. When you have the urge to eat, but you're not hungry, pay attention to how much mental and emotional discomfort you feel by not indulging. The results will tell you if you have become overly dependent on food for stress management. Adjust accordingly. Journal your thoughts and emotions.

Journal...

_____

_____

_____

_____

_____

_____

_____

_____

_____

_____

_____

_____

_____

Manage Your Time

"Let our advance worrying become advance thinking and planning." – Winston Churchill

To-Do's		Long-Term Goals
✔		☐
✔		☐
✔		☐
✔		☐
✔		☐
✔		☐
✔		☐
✔		☐
✔		☐
✔		☐
✔		☐

I don't include the Churchill quote to tell you to worry—there's enough worry to go around. Focus on the words "advance thinking and planning." This tip plays into some of the others which have dealt with procrastination and living in the moment.

Time is the ultimate unrenewable resource. **The next minute you live is the last time you will live that minute.** The best question we can often ask is, "How do I make the most of my time?' We need to know a couple of things to answer this accurately. First: What do I want? Where do I want to be? What do I wish was different? These are questions that you can only answer with a study of how you spend your time.

And that's the other thing we need to know. *How do I spend my time?* The only way to really put this in perspective is to track it. You probably have more time than you think. At the very least, you probably spend some time on activities that don't contribute to your goals, and you don't even realize how often it happens, or how many minutes are squandered.

Commitment: Get a daily planner. Use it for a month. Give yourself a chance to document *exactly* how you spend your time. Don't let a planner micromanage you like a tyrant, but give yourself a chance to see just how you're allocating your minutes. You'll know what to do next.

Journal...

_____
_____
_____
_____
_____
_____
_____
_____
_____
_____
_____
_____
_____
_____
_____
_____
_____
_____

Keep In Touch With Family

"You don't choose your family. They are God's gift to you, as you are to them." – Desmond Tutu

To-Do's		Long-Term Goals

Even if you don't believe in God as Desmond Tutu does, you can admit that you didn't get to choose your family. And if you were raised by your parents, and alongside your siblings, here is a simple fact: **the adult you are is largely the product of those years in which you were being raised.** And the people who were closest to you at that time have inestimable influence over the rest of your future.

If you are lucky enough to have a good family that you love, you won a lottery ticket. Your family will always be there for you. Your family will always love you. It's impossible for them to stop. You will always have their support. They will always find a way to forgive you. They will always be there to listen.

And these are the things you owe them as well. Your family should be full of the most loving relationships of your life. Nurture these relationships. Never let them go. You won't have them forever.

Commitment: This week, make contact with everyone in your family. Commit to doing this at least once a week.

Journal...

Brush And Floss

"The man with a toothache thinks everyone happy whose teeth are sound. The poverty-stricken man makes the same mistake about the rich man." – George Bernard Shaw

To-Do's		Long-Term Goals
✔	Life comes with a lot of toil and tasks. There are so many things to do each day that would be sheer drudgery if we stopped to think about them. But ignoring the small tasks, even something like daily brushing and flossing, can have major consequences.	☐
✔		☐
✔	Yes, even though brushing and flossing is a brief task, over the years, a staggering amount of time is lost to the simple act of scrubbing your teeth so they don't rot out of your head, and running a strip of floss between them so that your gums will be healthy.	☐
✔		☐
✔	Consider the alternative. The pain of toothaches, lost teeth, the inability to concentrate that almost feels unique to tooth pain, and the clichéd but real anxiety of a trip to the dentist...**these things pale in comparison to the minute dedication it takes to practice basic dental hygiene.**	☐
✔		☐
✔		☐
✔	**Commitment:** Brush at least three times a day. Floss every day. Make this a ritual. No excuses, no exceptions.	☐

Journal...

Understand Depression

"Depression is the inability to construct a future." – Rollo May

To-Do's		Long-Term Goals
✔		☐
✔		☐
✔		☐
✔		☐
✔		☐
✔		☐
✔		☐
✔		☐
✔		☐

If you've never experienced depression, it can be confusing. It might not even look real. It's tempting to think of depression as just being really, really, *really* sad, and who hasn't experienced sadness, right? But until you've experienced the agony of real, diagnosable depression, you just don't know what you don't know. Depression is real. It is as real as a sprained ankle.

The Depression and Bipolar Support Alliance estimates that nearly fifteen million people in America alone are suffering from acute depression. The numbers are certainly higher than that, as not all cases are reported or treated.

If you can believe these numbers, you can see how a better understanding of depression will aid you in your practice of empathy and compassion. **Chances are you know, or love, someone who has or will suffer from depression.** The more you know, the better of a support you'll be able to be.

Commitment: Read *The Noonday Demon: An Atlas of Depression* by Andrew Solomon. It's a beautiful, readable book book about a devastating subject, and is the best introduction to the subject.

Journal...

_____
_____
_____
_____
_____
_____
_____
_____
_____
_____
_____
_____
_____
_____
_____
_____
_____
_____
_____
_____

Be Assertive

"I need to learn to be more assertive." – Brooke Elliott, Broadway Star

To-Do's		Long-Term Goals

To be assertive, you need to know what you want from your life, and how you expect other people to treat you. Being assertive is more than simply standing up for yourself, and it's not just a form of contrarianism. You don't need to play Devil's advocate in every conversation just to feel like you asserted yourself, or included yourself.

Real, practicable, personal, useful assertiveness is about self-respect. It is about confidence. It can look overly forceful to people who are not assertive, and if you're not careful, you can overdo it and turn an attempt at assertiveness into something excessive and bullying.

When practicing assertiveness, simply keep the following foundations in mind: kindness, compassion, empathy. If you stick to those bedrocks while asserting yourself, you have no reason to regret or doubt the results. Speak up and get yourself the life you want. Control what you can control. You deserve to be treated well, heard, respected, and loved. If you do not teach people how to treat you, they may never learn.

Commitment: If you're a people pleaser, spend this week trying to think less about people's reactions to your words and actions, and have a conversation that you have been avoiding.

Journal...

April

Look Around And Pay Attention

"You can always find a distraction if you're looking for one." – Tom Kite

To-Do's

- ✔
- ✔
- ✔
- ✔
- ✔
- ✔
- ✔
- ✔
- ✔

Long-Term Goals

- ☐
- ☐
- ☐
- ☐
- ☐
- ☐
- ☐
- ☐
- ☐

Take a walk today and you'll probably see the same thing as everyone else who's out for a walk today. People staring at or talking on their phones, listening to music as they walk, and basically, not paying attention. This will rarely have a negative consequence beyond annoying the luddites around you who mourn the continued presence of technology.

But ask yourself an honest question. Do you pay attention as much as you used to when you're out with your gadgets? The answer is almost certainly no. When you didn't have a smartphone, you didn't go outside and stare at the ground, or your hand, while you walked. You paid attention. **And if you're not paying attention on this day, you might fall for some terrible hoaxes.**

Let's keep this very simple, with an easy example. Ask yourself if you still look both ways before you cross the street, just like you learned as a child. I hope so.

Commitment: Keep your head up when you're in public. You'll be safer from traffic, and you'll maintain an awareness of who is around you. Awareness is the first tenet of any basic self-defense course. Consider yourself warned.

Journal...

Narrate Your Environment

"The two most important things to do for self-defense are not to take a martial arts class or get a gun, but to think like the opposition and know where you're most at risk." – Barry Eisler

To-Do's		Long-Term Goals

Let's build off the previous tip. A lot of self-defense classes start with things like, "Here's how to get out of a headlock, or a choke." This is wrongheaded for lots of reasons, but first and foremost, it assumes that the violent act against you *will* happen. Practical self-defense is mental at the outset. The best fight is the one you *don't* get in.

The easiest and most immediate way to do this is, as mentioned before, to pay attention to what's around you. You'll know who's there, and you'll also see *who's looking at you.* **To understand the criminal's victim selection process, you simply have to know that the criminal is looking for the sure thing, the least hassle.** Is it easy to knock someone on the head and take their wallet if they're looking up, or looking down at a phone? Obvious.

Here's an easy exercise to get in the habit of. As you're out, start a simple narration of what you see. It can be as basic as a word or two per glance. *Man in coat. Woman with stroller. Dog. Red Car With Black Top.* If you do this enough, you'll know when odd things are repeating themselves. If *Red car with black top* comes up four times in an hour, you might have someone paying you an undue amount of attention.

Commitment: Do not think of this as paranoia. It's always better to err on the side of caution when it comes to safety. Take a week to practice this narrative habit. It'll keep your head up and your attention focused. You'll be safer, and you'll present yourself as a less easy target.

Journal...

Stop Smoking

"Giving up smoking is the easiest thing in the world. I know because I've done it thousands of times." – Mark Twain

To-Do's		Long-Term Goals

To-Do's
- ✔
- ✔
- ✔
- ✔
- ✔
- ✔
- ✔
- ✔

The Center For Disease Control And Prevention estimates, as of 2015, that smoking still kills upwards of 480,000 people. Smoking is the largest cause of preventable death in America. This means that half a million people in the United States alone did not need to die from smoking-related complications. *(CDC 2015, Cigarette Smoking In The United States)*

There's just not much more to say. Smoking causes cancer, it gives you bad breath, it ruins your teeth, it wrecks your lungs, it's a bad example for kids, you have to go outside in the cold to smoke, and the list goes on and on.

For those of you who believe it's hard to stop, **the truth is it's actually harder to smoke than *not* to smoke.** If you smoke, you must plan ahead. You must always be prepared. If you don't smoke, then you just don't smoke.

Commitment: Stop smoking. Every medical aid you need to stop is actually sold over the counter now. If you don't smoke, don't start. Ever.

Long-Term Goals
- ☐
- ☐
- ☐
- ☐
- ☐
- ☐
- ☐
- ☐

Journal...

Be Honest About Your Vices And Habits

"Men are more easily governed through their vices than through their virtues." – Napoleon Bonaparte

To-Do's		Long-Term Goals
✔	One of the greatest gifts we can give ourselves is the freedom to make choices. This might sound simplistic, but consider the previous tip about smoking. People who die of smoking-related complications are making the choice to smoke, sure, but they are not as free as they could be. Something else is influencing their choices, if not making them outright. Ultimately, they will experience a physical prison of their choices, whether it's a chronic cough, inability to run, or the persistent need for oxygen.	☐
✔		☐
✔		☐
✔		☐
✔	If you are dependent on a substance or sensation, whether it's alcohol, nicotine, tea, junk food, sex, adrenaline, etc, you are not as free as you could be. **With the loss of freedom, any amount of freedom, comes the loss of choice.** There is no autonomy in compulsion.	☐
✔		☐
✔	The clearest way to think about it is this: Today, do you have to *choose* whether to drink, smoke, chew tobacco, eat a Twinkie, or anything similar? If you have to *think* about it, you're verging on a compulsion, a deep-set habit that you might not have as much control over as you think. If you're not doing it simply because you enjoy it, if you would experience some agitation if you went without, there are questions to ask yourself about your vice.	☐
✔		☐
✔		☐
✔	**Commitment:** Abstain from a substance or sensation for one week that you think you might be dependent on. Write down your experience, particularly noting if you get irritable or have physical symptoms in the absence of your habit.	☐
✔		☐
✔		☐

Journal...

_____

_____

_____

_____

_____

_____

_____

_____

_____

_____

_____

_____

_____

_____

_____

_____

Get A Physical

"I mean some doctor told me I had six months to live and I went to their funeral." – Keith Richards

To-Do's		Long-Term Goals

✔

✔

✔

✔

✔

✔

✔

No matter how well we take care of ourselves, in the end, our bodies will eventually give in to time and age. **Our bodies are not immortal.** What we do have control over is the way we care for our bodies.

But no matter how much you exercise, or how on-point your nutrition is, you will never know everything that is happening inside you. You need a professional to check you out, and this becomes more important as you age.

You don't want to turn into a hypochondriac and rush to the ER every time you catch a cold, but at the very least, you should get a physical each year. There are countless stories of people who caught the early spread of a disease, even something as insidious as cancer, just because they went in for a routine check up.

Commitment: Schedule a physical. Go to the appointment. Schedule the next physical while you're there, even if it's a year away.

☐ ☐ ☐ ☐ ☐ ☐ ☐

Journal...

Write A Thank You Note

"'Thank you' is the best prayer that anyone could say. I say that one a lot. Thank you expresses extreme gratitude, humility, understanding." – Alice Walker

To-Do's		Long-Term Goals

Think about how good it feels to receive a sincere "thank you" from someone you have touched. Part of the poignancy of it is that, when you truly move someone, you don't always hear about it right away. **Getting thanked for something you'd forgotten you even did can be like a present showing up when it's not your birthday.**

Now, think about the people you could thank. There are probably plenty of them. Teachers, parents, siblings, friends, co-workers, authors, filmmakers, the guy at the hot dog stand who always smiles, a crossing guard who holds a stop sign for kids on even the coldest mornings...so many other people can make a difference if we pay enough attention to notice.

Why not write one of them a thank you note? You'll feel good and so will they. You don't even have to do it in person, just mail it, drop it off somewhere where they will find it, or have someone deliver it anonymously. There's added charm to a handwritten note these days.

Commitment: Write a thank you note this week. It can be to anyone you want, just give it to someone you feel genuine gratitude for.

Journal...

Make Someone Else Look Good

"Sometimes, whether you like it or not, people elevate you. It's real easy to fall." – Eddie Vedder

To-Do's
✔
✔
✔
✔
✔
✔
✔
✔

Long-Term Goals
☐
☐
☐
☐
☐
☐
☐
☐

This tip works particularly well if you know someone who is struggling, someone who feels abandoned, or someone who is legitimately being ignored. An obvious place to make someone look good is at work, when reputations and performance dictate the rate at which one can make progress.

This can be as simple as complimenting someone in front of other people, giving genuine, honest praise to work well done, inviting someone to lunch with you who seems to have a hard time fitting into the group...there is no shortage of options.

Of course, putting the spotlight on someone else means that it is off of you for the moment. If you're always craving attention, this can be a great way to work on two goals at once--freeing yourself of the need for validation, and elevating someone else in the process.

Commitment: Pick someone you see regularly. Think of a way to sing their praises to others. Do it, and see how happy a small, thoughtful act can make someone else.

Journal...

_____
_____
_____
_____
_____
_____
_____
_____
_____
_____
_____
_____
_____
_____
_____
_____
_____
_____
_____
_____
_____
_____

Don't Stay At A Job Your Hate

"Instead of wondering when your next vacation is, maybe you should set up a life you don't need to escape from." – Seth Godin

To-Do's

- ✔
- ✔
- ✔
- ✔
- ✔
- ✔
- ✔
- ✔
- ✔
- ✔
- ✔

Long-Term Goals

- ☐
- ☐
- ☐
- ☐
- ☐
- ☐
- ☐
- ☐
- ☐
- ☐
- ☐

Most of us spend so much of our lives working. Someone has to pay the bills, and I doubt anyone is beating down your door to pay yours. So we go to work. **We sell our time in exchange for a paycheck.** We make ends meet, we take our vacations, hopefully we like what we're doing, and this is just the way it usually goes.

But sometimes we have jobs that we hate. That are literally bad for us. Toxic environments, domineering bosses, jobs with such low pay that we can't meet our financial responsibilities, and more. There are many ways that a job can go wrong. And a job that you hate, given the amount of time you will spend there, is not worth keeping.

It's terrifying to think about leaving a job when money is tight, or even when it's not. Once you've invested a certain amount of time in a place, leaving can make the years feels wasted. What about the 401K? Insurance? Where's my paycheck going to come from next?

But life is short. It's clichéd but true. There are a lot of jobs out there. You might even love some of them. This is one area where having passions can really help give you guidance.

Commitment: If you hate your job, find a way to leave it or a way to improve it. Start by improving yourself. Ask, What can I be doing better at my job? You deserve to be happy, and not just at work.

Journal...

_____

_____

_____

_____

_____

_____

_____

_____

_____

_____

_____

_____

_____

_____

_____

_____

_____

_____

Eliminate Toxic People From Your Life

"Toxic people attach themselves like cinder blocks tied to your ankles, and then invite you for a swim in their poisoned waters." – John Green

To-Do's		Long-Term Goals

Let's define the term first. A person is not toxic in, say, the same way that arsenic is toxic. A toxic person exhibits toxic behavior, or it is your relationship with the person that is toxic.

Being around a toxic person leaves you feeling depleted, not energized. You might dread being around them. They might make you feel ashamed, or even speak abusively to you. Toxic people are generally manipulative and domineering. They might make the conversations all about them and you wind up feeling like you're nothing but an audience.

But the main thing to pay attention to is the energy that a person takes out of you. Whether or not you label them toxic isn't the point. You need to end relationships with people who put less into the relationship than they add.

Commitment: Eliminating toxic people from your life can be tricky. They can be emotionally volatile, very persuasive, and might try to convince you that you're wrong, or that they can change. If you think they deserve another chance, set boundaries. Make your expectations clear. Stick to the plan when and if they break your trust.

Journal...

Make Aging With Dignity A Goal

"My issue isn't about physical aging; my issue is about wanting to remain vigorous and youthful in my spirit." –
Rob Lowe

To-Do's		Long-Term Goals

Unawares, a day will arrive when you have more days behind you than in front of you. In the second half of our lives, our fitness priorities and goals may shift. No matter how committed you are, it will not always be possible to put on more muscle, to jump higher, to run further. There is a day when our physical limitations will dictate what our goals must be.

Others might persuade you that there is no more noble goal than simply aging well. Meaning, age without pain. Age without decreased mobility. Age without weight gain and a loss of bone density. True, a simple, regular exercise routine will give you an elevated quality of life in your later years. But did you come this far just to not hurt?

Your goal, instead, is to Age with dignity. Age with wisdom. Age with standing. Age with compassion and kindness. Age like the life you have left matters.

And this is true regardless of your current age, since you will never know when you crossed that halfway mark.

Commitment: If you are not elderly, start, or continue, with your exercise regimen. If you are a senior citizen, see a doctor, get their recommendations for an exercise program that will help you maximize your physical potential at this stage. If you are wise, you will cultivate dignity, patience, compassion, and kindness.

Journal...

_____

_____

_____

_____

_____

_____

_____

_____

_____

_____

_____

_____

_____

_____

_____

_____

_____

Donate Your Books

"There are worse crimes than burning books. One of them is not reading them." – Ray Bradbury

To-Do's

✔

✔

✔

✔

✔

✔

✔

✔

Many people can't afford to buy every book they read, and even those who can may not have enough space to store them all. But once you've read the book, there it is, sitting on the shelf. If you suspect that you're never going to read it again, and you would like to free up the space, consider donating it. **Share the joy.**

Many thrift stores sell books for less than two dollars. Most libraries will consider donations as well, provided that they fill a need in the library collection. And many, particularly those that are underfunded, may be extremely grateful for the generous act.

Passing a book onward, even if you can't profit from it by selling it, means that someone else may get a chance to be enriched by it. If you've ever loved a book, you know what that can mean.

Commitment: Rather than discarding your books or letting them pile up to a level of clutter that bothers you, consider donating them after reading.

Long-Term Goals

☐

☐

☐

☐

☐

☐

☐

☐

Journal...

Consider A Pet

"He who is cruel to animals becomes hard also in his dealings with men. We can judge the heart of a man by his treatment of animals." – Immanuel Kant

To-Do's		Long-Term Goals

✔

✔

✔

✔

✔

✔

✔

✔

One of the easiest ways to ensure that you get a little bit of exercise each day—or several times a day—is to get a dog that needs to be walked. This might seem like an extreme way to go about it, but there are plenty of other reasons to consider getting a pet.

People who aren't animal lovers might sneer at the idea that an animal can make you feel loved, or that enjoying an animal's devotion is something pitiful. But we are focused on results here, and if a pet makes you happier, no one else's opinion should matter.

Research has also shown that pets can increase allergy resistance, lower heart rate by acting as stress relieving mechanisms, and more. **Rescuing an animal from certain euthanasia is a soul-healing experience that is very powerful.**

Commitment: Visit a rescue shelter. Check out the animals. If any of them tug at your heartstrings, you may have found a friend that will appreciate you for as long as you're together.

☐ ☐ ☐ ☐ ☐ ☐ ☐ ☐

Journal...

Cry If You Need To

"Why is it you feel like a dope if you laugh alone, but that's usually how you end up crying?" – Chuck Palahniuk

To-Do's		Long-Term Goals

Wellness doesn't have a gender, but crying is too often seen only as the province of women. Catharsis does not have a gender either, and few things can be as cleansing—in that I-Just-Hit-The-Reset-Button-Way—as a good cry.

But consider this, especially if you're a man. When you have a strong emotion like anger, what do you do? You probably don't fight against the anger with all your might, as if releasing it would be a failure or a shame. Why would you try to hold it in when you feel the urge to cry just as strongly? **Is there any way to pretend that this tamping down of the impulse doesn't come with a cost?**

If you think you are too tough to cry, you are denying yourself the reset button.

Commitment: Don't fight it. Just cry when you have to. Don't think of it as admitting failure or weakness, but rather a reset button.

Journal...

From Tolerance To Acceptance

"I have seen great intolerance shown in support of tolerance." – Samuel Taylor Coleridge

To-Do's		Long-Term Goals

There are two parts to this one, and part one is a question. **Is tolerance a virtue?** Before you answer, think about this carefully. When you hear that someone tolerates a thing, what you're usually hearing is someone saying "I don't like it, I don't want it, and this is the closest I can come to not flat out saying I hate it."

Think about someone "tolerating" the fact that a person you love dearly is gay, or Chinese, or female, or male, or Christian, or Muslim, or Republican or Democrat. Tolerance no longer sounds like such a generous word.

Part two: Most people seem to think that tolerance is the same thing as acceptance. It's not. This doesn't mean you should accept or condone actions or viewpoints that you find reprehensible. You should neither "tolerate" nor "accept" something like racism. But be honest with yourself. Do you tolerate, or do you practice true acceptance?

Commitment: Define tolerance for yourself. Then, think about whether you are tolerating things in others that you could actually accept, if not full-on embrace.

Journal...

Pay Your Taxes

"The avoidance of taxes is the only intellectual pursuit that still carries any reward." – John Maynard Keynes

To-Do's
✔
✔
✔
✔
✔
✔
✔

Tax season comes around every year, like it or not. Even if you don't have an exotic financial situation, filing taxes can be a daunting task, and the fear of getting it wrong can make the whole process a misery, even when it goes well.

One of the greatest gifts for your peace of mind is to learn how your taxes work, and to keep track of all extra income during the year. If you **start a spreadsheet** and get into the habit of logging all extra income, you'll have everything that you—or a tax preparation expert—will need in order to file accurately and efficiently.

Avoid filing an extension for your taxes unless absolutely necessary. It might free up some headspace in the short-term, but it can also be easy to forget for another year, or to let it slide. Then the situation is more complicated.

Commitment: Learn how your taxes work. File them quickly and efficiently every year.

Long-Term Goals
☐
☐
☐
☐
☐
☐
☐

Journal...

_____
_____
_____
_____
_____
_____
_____
_____
_____
_____
_____
_____
_____
_____
_____
_____
_____
_____
_____
_____
_____
_____
_____

Sing!

"If you see the sunset, does it have to mean something? If you hear the birds singing does it have to have a message?" – Robert Wilson

To-Do's		Long-Term Goals
✔	If you observe a group of children at a park or playground, the chances are high that you'll witness at least a few of them bursting into song at random intervals. Why? Well, that's the wrong question. Ask instead, *Hmm, what do they know that I don't?*	☐
✔		☐
✔	When was the last time you sang because, well, you just had to sing? When you couldn't stand not to do a little dance and invent a little melody to accompany your adventures that day?	☐
✔		☐
✔	You don't have to be Whitney Houston to enjoy singing. It makes you feel *good*. It doesn't matter if you've got a decent "choir" voice that's perfect for blending, or you croak like a demented, off-key toad. **Enthusiastic singing is perhaps the greatest example of the absence of self-consciousness.**	☐
✔		☐
✔		☐
✔	**Commitment:** Sometime this week, when you're alone if need be, just pick a song and belt it out from start to finish. You'll probably end up smiling, or at least notice something worth smiling about.	☐

Journal...

_____
_____
_____
_____
_____
_____
_____
_____
_____
_____
_____
_____
_____
_____
_____
_____
_____
_____
_____
_____

Be A Better Kisser

"Any man who can drive safely while kissing a pretty girl is simply not giving the kiss the attention it deserves."
– Albert Einstein

To-Do's		Long-Term Goals

According to *Time* magazine, psychologist John Bohannon from Butler University has found that most of us can recall up to 90 percent of the details of a first romantic kiss. In his study of five hundred people, most remembered this experience more vividly than their first sexual encounter.

Why would this be? Well, **kissing feels good**, it's often a prelude to something more arousing, and there may be biological factors in play. From *The Science of Kissing: What Our Lips Are Telling us,* "59% of men and 66% of women have ended a relationship because someone was a bad kisser." Now, bad can mean many things—bad breath, bad technique, *or* bad indicator that a long-term, romantic, procreative relationship (remember, we're talking biological precedents)—but not many people want to stay with someone if the kissing is never going to be great.

Commitment: Read *The Science of Kissing* and see how you measure up to the author's data. Have fun and keep practicing.

Journal...

Limit Social Media Time

"Social media is an amazing tool, but it's really the face-to-face interaction that makes a long-term impact." –
Felicia Day

To-Do's

- ✔
- ✔
- ✔
- ✔
- ✔
- ✔
- ✔
- ✔
- ✔

Long-Term Goals

☐
☐
☐
☐
☐
☐
☐
☐

The rise of social media has made it easier to connect with friends, stay in touch with family, share your own experiences, and more. It can also make it much easier to waste time, and in some ways, it has changed the nature of experience itself.

Scroll through a Facebook feed and you might ask yourself this question: Is the point of going on a hike to go on a hike, or to share a photo of going on a hike? Ditto for going to a concert, eating a meal, having a drink with a friend, etc. You can get the impression quickly that an experience not worth sharing is not worth having. You can also start to think that none of us ever have a thought that goes unshared.

Social media can become a compulsion, and like all compulsions, it can diminish our ability to choose. Taking a step back from time to time can be a healthy way to reevaluate how your social media time may be affecting your life.

Commitment: Read *You Are Not A Gadget* by Jaron Lanier. Try spending today off of social media.

Journal...

_____
_____
_____
_____
_____
_____
_____
_____
_____
_____
_____
_____
_____
_____
_____
_____
_____
_____
_____
_____

Be Polite

"Politeness is a desire to be treated politely, and to be esteemed polite oneself." – Francois de la Rouchefoucauld

To-Do's		Long-Term Goals

It is so easy to be polite to people, unless you've gotten out of the habit, or never developed it to begin with. But why would it be important? "I don't care what people think" or "I'm not changing who I am for anyone" are familiar refrains from people who prefer to see their rudeness as assertiveness and authenticity.

A question worth asking: **Can you actually see a downside to being polite?** I suspect not, unless your definitions are muddled. If you think that treating others respectfully makes you a doormat or a people pleaser, sure, I can see how you'd give politeness a bad rap. But you're just not looking at it in the most helpful way.

There's no downside to being polite. Not when it comes to true politeness. At the very least, surely we can all admit that there's no upside to blatant rudeness.

Commitment: This week, be more polite than you feel. At the very least, avoid all forms of rudeness. See if you notice a difference in the way you feel, and in the way that people interact with you.

Journal...

Improve Your Vocabulary

"One forgets words as one forgets names. One's vocabulary needs constant fertilizing or it will die." – Evelyn Waugh

To-Do's		Long-Term Goals

✔

✔

✔

✔

✔

✔

✔

✔

✔

You've probably known someone with a showy vocabulary. Someone who trots out a five syllable word when a one syllable word would have done. But this shouldn't distort your perceptions of just how useful an ever-expanding vocabulary can be.

Most importantly, much of thought takes place in language. I'm not talking about images and memories. Think about trying to follow a complex argument, or formulating one, or trying to familiarize yourself with a concept you've never heard of. **Words are the tools of your understanding.** They are also the audible manifestations of your internal thoughts. In this way, your ability to comprehend as much as possible hinges on your facility with language.

There are few gifts you can give your brain that will serve it as well as a mastery of language.

Commitment: Sign up for one of the many Vocabulary Word Of The Day sites online. A new word will arrive for you every day. Start using the word as soon as you can. It'll help you retain it.

☐ ☐ ☐ ☐ ☐ ☐ ☐ ☐ ☐

Journal...

Practice Compassion, Not Pity

"Three passions, simple but overwhelmingly strong, have governed my life: the longing for love, the search for knowledge, and unbearable pity for the suffering of mankind." – Bertrand Russell

To-Do's
✓
✓
✓
✓
✓
✓
✓
✓
✓

Compassion literally means to be able to suffer along with someone else. To put yourself in their shoes and imagine how they must be feeling. But when you hear someone say they felt compassion for someone, they're often describing something closer to pity, and nobody wants to be pitied.

If you hear someone say, "Oh, I feel so sorry for him." You're not really hearing compassion here. You're hearing pity. You're not necessarily speaking with someone practicing compassion, you're hearing someone who is also thinking *I'm glad that's not happening to me.* This distance is the opposite of real compassion.

But acknowledging that someone is experiencing something painful does not get you closer to being able to help them. Long-term pity is more likely to produce distaste than anything. **Compassion leads to solutions and empathy.** Know the difference.

Commitment: The next time someone close to you is suffering, ask yourself if you know the difference between compassion and pity. How good are you at putting yourself in their shoes? The better you are at it, the more likely that you will be able to offer the kind of support they'll need the most.

Long-Term Goals
☐
☐
☐
☐
☐
☐
☐
☐
☐

Journal...

_____
_____
_____
_____
_____
_____
_____
_____
_____
_____
_____
_____
_____
_____
_____
_____
_____
_____

Read With A Dictionary

"Always read something that will make you look good if you die in the middle of it." – P.J. O'Rourke

To-Do's

- ✔
- ✔
- ✔
- ✔
- ✔
- ✔
- ✔
- ✔
- ✔

Back in school, you may have been taught to read past an unfamiliar word and try to learn its meaning from context. This is a good strategy when learning words is the goal. But it can work at cross purposes if you find yourself *finishing* fewer books than you would like to.

Now, if you skip one word and its meaning never becomes clear to you, you can probably soldier on without it taking much of a toll. But if you do this over and over, there's an accumulating mental fatigue that will wear your brain out and make you stop sooner than you might have.

If you know the feeling of brain-deadness while reading, it could actually be because you are encountering too many words that you don't know, and the reading part of your brain wants to stop because it can't comprehend much of what you're doing.

Commitment: When you read, read with a dictionary. Look up words you don't know. E-readers like the Kindle now have dictionaries built into them, making it even easier. Even if it seems cumbersome, the sooner you start, the less often you'll have to refer to a dictionary in the future.

Long-Term Goals

- ☐
- ☐
- ☐
- ☐
- ☐
- ☐
- ☐
- ☐
- ☐

Journal...

_____
_____
_____
_____
_____
_____
_____
_____
_____
_____
_____
_____
_____
_____
_____
_____
_____
_____
_____
_____

Don't Take Offense

"We should be too big to take offense and too noble to give it." – Abraham Lincoln

To-Do's		Long-Term Goals

✔

✔

✔

✔

✔

✔

✔

✔

When people say, "That offends me," they often think they have made an argument, or a point. But all they have done is acknowledge that they are now offended. I'm sure you've been offended before. Clichés persist because there is truth in them, and one perennial cliché is that being offended is a choice.

Do you believe this? The theory is sound, although in practice it is much harder. When someone says something that makes your blood boil, good luck turning it off immediately! **But you do have control over the next choice you make.** Will you yell? Argue? Storm out of the room? Tell everyone you know about how horribly you were treated? Quit your job? Throw office supplies until your poor Human Resources manager fires you?

Like it or not, no matter how wronged you have been, only you can control what you do in the aftermath.

Commitment: The next time you feel offended, think and breathe before responding. Tell yourself that you choose not to be offended. See if it helps.

☐ ☐ ☐ ☐ ☐ ☐ ☐

Journal...

Don't One-Up People

"When boasting ends, there dignity begins." – Owen D. Young

To-Do's	Long-Term Goals

You've probably seen this scenario unfold more than once. Someone – maybe you – tells a story. It's funny, or interesting, or sad, but it's *compelling* and everyone knows it. And then, the story reminds someone else of something that happened to them, and it's even funnier, or more interesting, or sadder, and more compelling. It takes the focus off of the first storyteller and has a deflating effect.

We all know a one-upper. **Maybe we've all been one at times.** But it's a tedious, indecorous trait that never looks good. There is enough room for everyone to tell their stories, and we all have them. Just because someone tells a great story doesn't mean that you're *not* interesting. You don't have to prove it.

Just sit back, enjoy other people's tales, and add your own when it makes sense to do so.

Commitment: Don't be a one-upper. Save your own great stories for a time when they can receive the full spotlight they deserve.

Journal...

Learn A New Language

"If you talk to a man in a language he understands, that goes to his head. If you talk to him in his own language, that goes to his heart." – Nelson Mandela

To-Do's		Long-Term Goals

Most of us were required to take a foreign language class in high school. And for most of us, the chances that the one year of high school French or Spanish made us (and kept us) fluent is almost precisely zero. We learn to speak whatever our native language is as a child, but it is never too late to learn a new one, no matter what people say about old dogs and new tricks.

Because learning a language isn't a trick. It is actually quite simple, it just takes dedication, time, and practice. The benefits of learning a new language include: greater potential ease while traveling in a foreign country, flexing a part of your brain that your native language doesn't touch, being able to discover new authors and singers in foreign languages, and so much more. **Learning a language is like putting together a puzzle that both expands your horizons and rewards you for the rest of your life.**

Commitment: Download the program Duolingo and sign up (it's free) for the language of your choice. You can make great progress in even 10 minutes a day, as long as you stick with it.

Journal...

You Know Enough To Train Yourself

"If a man achieves victory over this body, who in the world can exercise power over him? He who rules himself rules over the whole world." – Vinoba Bhave

To-Do's
✔
✔
✔
✔
✔
✔
✔
✔
✔
✔
✔
✔

The fitness industry makes its money by increasing the perception of the knowledge gap between the trainer and the trainee. It makes more money if it can convince you that you have no idea what you should do with your own fitness and that you need to be dependent on "experts."

Granted, if someone with little to no experience walks into a modern gym that is furnished with 50 million machines and options, they might not know where to start. The truth is, they could start with a space no larger than a phone booth and make great progress for years if they were patient and focused on the basics. Lift challenging weights. Use big, compound movements if you can do so without pain. Sleep enough. Rinse and repeat.

This is not to dismiss the invaluable contributions of elite physiologists and sports scientists and elite trainers who specialize in Athletic Performance. However, most people aren't looking for a trainer to make them elite. They want to be healthier. To lose the last 10 pounds. To learn safe technique.

The problem with relying on someone else is that it could take away from the formation of your habits. If you NEED your trainer, what do you do when your trainer moves away, or gets fired, or he takes another job? At that point, if you feel lost, then your trainer has not done his job.

Commitment: If you are interested in general fitness, muscle gain, fat loss, like most people...you will eventually need to know enough to do the job for yourself. Ask more questions about proper lifting form and mechanics. Read *4 Hour Body* by Tim Ferris.

Long-Term Goals
☐
☐
☐
☐
☐
☐
☐
☐
☐
☐
☐
☐

Journal...

_____

_____

_____

_____

_____

_____

_____

_____

_____

_____

_____

Know Your Why

"There is a plan and a purpose, a value to every life, no matter what its location, age, gender or disability." – Sharron Angle

To-Do's		Long-Term Goals

Why do you get up in the morning? Why do you go to work? Why do you pursue the hobbies that you do? Why do you spend time with friends, or choose not to? Why get married? Why start a family? Why why why?

It's easy to answer many of these questions with, "Because it's what people do" or "What else would I do?" But there is a better answer, and it comes down to knowing your "why." Think about what you want to accomplish with your life. "Going through the motions and then dying," is not a response you would give, even if that's what your actions might look like to an outside observer.

In order to have a purpose, you have to know what it is. **Only you can give your life meaning.** In order to know what your purpose is, you have to think about it and really put in the hard work of contemplation. Once you know what your "why" is, you can then measure all of your decisions and actions against it.

Commitment: Pretend that tomorrow morning someone is going to stop you and say, "Hey, what's your Why?" Have an answer for them. Youtube Jim Rohn's video on 4 Questions to Ponder.

Journal...

You Might Not Need All That Cardio

"I always find cardio the most monotonous. Running on a treadmill shows me why hamsters are so crazy." – Luke Evans

To-Do's

✔

✔

✔

✔

✔

✔

✔

✔

Long-Term Goals

☐

☐

☐

☐

☐

☐

☐

☐

The word cardio generally brings up images of people on treadmills, elliptical machines, rowers, or Stairmasters. And these things can all be great, depending on what your goals are. However, it's important to remember that what we mean by "cardio" usually just refers to getting our heartrates elevated in order to increase our conditioning levels or to get into a fat-burning zone.

But there are a lot of ways to get your heart rate up. You could simply lift weights faster, or give yourself shorter rests in between. You can jump rope or do sprints in a swimming pool. Kettlebell training provides fast, ballistic movements that can deliver the fat-loss results of a treadmill without the monotony.

If you like cardio, traditional cardio, by all means, stick with it. If you've ever wished there was a better way, you have more options than you might be aware of.

Commitment: If you're sick of traditional cardio, experiment with anything mentioned above, or get creative and come up with something on your own. Just focus on your heart rate.

Journal...

_____
_____
_____
_____
_____
_____
_____
_____
_____
_____
_____
_____
_____
_____
_____
_____
_____
_____
_____
_____

Study Multiple Religions

"I have been all things unholy. If God can work through me, he can work through anyone." – Francis of Assisi

To-Do's

- ✔
- ✔
- ✔
- ✔
- ✔
- ✔
- ✔
- ✔

Religion can offer invaluable peace and direction for some, even as others associate it with unimaginable strife and destruction. **But at the root of religion—all religions and denominations—is the search for happiness and guidance.**

One way to avoid the schisms and infighting among the many sects is to study multiple, many, or all religions. In this way, you will see how they are alike, how they are different, and have access to new questions that will give you the ability to think more clearly about religion as a whole.

If nothing else, few things are as fascinating as The Big Questions, and religion, regardless of whether you think it successfully provides answers or not, concerns itself primarily with the big picture.

Commitment: Read about the beliefs of another church. Start with Kadampa Buddhism, a branch of Buddhism whose main purpose is to attain world peace. That's one mission I can get behind regardless of my personal beliefs.

Long-Term Goals

- ☐
- ☐
- ☐
- ☐
- ☐
- ☐
- ☐
- ☐

Journal...

What's Your Story?

"Tell the truth, or someone will tell it for you." – Stephanie Klein

To-Do's		Long-Term Goals

✔

✔

✔

✔

✔

✔

✔

✔

✔

Pretend that you've just been offered a memoir contract. You finally get the chance to tell your story. Only...do you know what it is? You probably thought you did. But if you actually sat down to write the story that you would want everyone else to know, do you have any idea what it would be? Or how you would go about it?

Where would you start? What events have been most pivotal in the shaping of your personality? Where do your beliefs comes from? Do you even have beliefs? What should you leave out? Who in your life has played the biggest supporting role? Do you have things to say about other people that might hurt you? Or them?

Let's scale down. What if someone said, "What's your story?" and you only had 30 seconds to tell them? What would you want them to know? **It's an elevator pitch of your life.**

Commitment: Really think about these questions. What's your story? Think about how you might answer it. If you really start feeling ambitious, try writing some of it down. You'll learn a lot about yourself.

☐ ☐ ☐ ☐ ☐ ☐ ☐ ☐ ☐

Journal...

May

Get A Bike

"Riding a bicycle is about getting back to basics. It's good for the waistline and it's good for the wallet..." – Phil Keoghan

To-Do's
✔
✔
✔
✔
✔
✔
✔

If you happen to live in an icy tundra where it is nothing but 24-7 blizzards, this tip might not be for you. For everyone else whose life includes the occasional dry road, it is time to get a bike. There are so many reasons to do it.

Riding a bike is cheaper than buying gas, and auto insurance, and auto inspection, and car washes, etc. It's also better for the environment. Commuting with a bike is also a great way to get some exercise. Driving a car isn't the most sedentary thing in the world, but it's a far cry from pedaling.

And whether every adult can admit it or not, riding a bike is fun. We knew this as kids. When people describe something as being, "Like riding a bike, you never forget," they're talking about the fun factor as well.

Commitment: Get a bike if you don't have one. Ride it regularly, not just for exercise, but also for fun.

Long-Term Goals
☐
☐
☐
☐
☐
☐
☐

Journal...

May 2

Be Healthy While Traveling

"A good traveler has no fixed plans, and is not intent on arriving." – Lao Tzu

To-Do's		Long-Term Goals
✔	With all due respect to Lao Tzu, there are some things worth planning for while traveling. Like fitness and healthy eating. It can be tough to get into a fitness routine, even under the best, most convenient circumstances, like when your gym is within walking distance of your house, and your kitchen's even closer.	☐
✔		☐
✔	If your trip is only a few days long, or even a week, there's nothing wrong with taking time off from eating well and working out, although it's certainly better to do *something* if you can. **Longer than a week and certain people can get derailed from the routine they were in, and herein lies the Traveling Trap.**	☐
✔		☐
✔		☐
✔	Before you take a trip, do a little planning. Plan on getting some exercise, even if it's pushups in the hotel room or laps in the pool. Go grocery shopping on your trip instead of eating out for every meal. Take some running shoes and go for a jog. Just putting out a little effort during the trip might mean you can pick right back up where you left off, once you're home again.	☐
✔		☐
✔		☐
✔	**Commitment:** The next time you travel, plan on making it the healthiest trip you've ever taken. Pack some workout clothes, even for a quick weekender.	☐

Journal...

_____

Clean Your House

"Life is denied by lack of attention, whether it be to cleaning windows or trying to write a masterpiece." – Nadia Boulanger

To-Do's		Long-Term Goals
✔	If I say to you, "It looks like a depressed person lives here," what do you picture? Probably a dim house full of clutter, dust, dishes in the sink, and a general sense of unkemptness. Why? Because keeping a clean house takes effort and diligence and energy, and these are exactly the things that get away from us when we're blue.	☐ ☐
✔		☐
✔	Now, there are plenty of happy, fulfilled people who don't have spotless houses. Namely, anyone with a child. **But beyond a certain point, a messy house hints at uncomfortable truths.** What does it mean if a clean environment is *not* a priority? Also, a messy house has a tendency to get messier still, if left untended.	☐
✔		☐
✔		☐
✔	Once you do a thorough deep cleaning of your house, you might find that it's easier to clear the clutter from your mind. Your creativity might soar. You might feel like you can breathe easier. And this is indisputable: it's easier to maintain a clean house than it is to deep clean one after it's gone too far.	☐
✔		☐
✔		☐
✔	**Commitment:** However tidy you are, commit to being cleaner. If you can, put something back in its place before leaving a room. Just form the habit. If you need help getting started, hire a maid for one day to do a deep cleaning. This could be as cheap as $50 for 4 hours of work.	☐
✔		☐

Journal...

_____
_____
_____
_____
_____
_____
_____
_____
_____
_____
_____
_____
_____
_____
_____
_____
_____
_____

Don't Brood

"I've always wanted to be a brooding, deep, dark artist, but I can never keep that facade going for more than 15 minutes." – Bryan Callen

To-Do's		Long-Term Goals

✔

✔

✔

✔

✔

✔

✔

✔

✔

If someone could observe you when you were alone, how would they describe you? Happy? Sleepy? Lazy? Sloppy? Brooding? Each of these descriptions would fit most of us at times. But let's focus on brooding. If you observe someone alone, and the person seems to be a brooder, what do you think you know about this person?

"Brooding" is often said in conjunction with the "strong, silent, type." What romance novels teach us is what every woman wants, not that brooding actually has a gender. But true brooding goes beyond being quiet or enigmatic. It is an immoderate amount of time spent in negative thought. **Brooding is the manifestation of a mind without enough room for light and levity.**

If you spend all of your time scowling and furrowing your brow, even if you're unaware of it, even if you're just in "deep thought," you're probably more likely to start to *think* like a brooding person with a furrowed brow.

Commitment: Brood when you must, but don't let it become your character. Try to be the person you would want someone to see, even when you're alone. Make room in your mind for levity.

☐ ☐ ☐ ☐ ☐ ☐ ☐ ☐ ☐

Journal...

_____
_____
_____
_____
_____
_____
_____
_____
_____
_____
_____
_____
_____
_____
_____
_____
_____
_____
_____

May 5

Eliminate "I Can't Believe This Is Happening"

"It takes courage to let go of the past and all the mechanisms you have put in place, in order to ease your pain, regret and fear through avoiding responsibility for it." – Shannon Alder

To-Do's

✔
✔
✔
✔
✔
✔
✔

Long-Term Goals

☐ ☐ ☐ ☐ ☐ ☐ ☐

Most crimes that involve a physical attack end within seven seconds. When the stakes are high—say, when a mugger jumps you in a parking lot at night—and things are suddenly moving fast, if you have time to think "I can't believe this is happening," it might already be too late.

But even if you're not in mortal danger, there are reasons to avoid thinking "I can't believe this is happening." Why? Because whatever "this," means to you in that moment, *it is happening.* And the sooner you can get from "I can't believe this is happening," to "This is happening," the sooner you can move on to "Now what?" which is all any of us truly have control over. **"What will happen next?" you get to control.**

Commitment: Whatever "This" is, when it's hard, tell yourself "This is happening." Then ask yourself, "What will I do next?" If you can form this habit, you'll bounce back from adversity quicker.

Journal...

Act Like A Kid (Sometimes)

"A little nonsense now and then, is cherished by the wisest men." – Roald Dahl

To-Do's		Long-Term Goals

There are plenty of childlike qualities that wouldn't serve us well in adult life. How would your boss react if you threw a tantrum the next time you were asked to do something you didn't want to do? Or you broke something just because you were curious about what would happen if you gave it a push?

But there are traits that we lose as adults that could work wonders on our well-being. A sense of playfulness. Enthusiasm. A wide-eyed curiosity about just how much there is to learn. Even the most intelligent of us will remain relatively childlike as far as the amount of knowledge we can amass. **We barely even know how much we *don't* know.**

Children are optimistic. Quick to forgive. They do not worry about yesterday or tomorrow as much as adults do.

Commitment: Reintroduce a sense of playfulness into your life. Reengage your child-like curiosity. Ask questions. Be persistent. Have fun.

Journal...

Eat Slowly. Especially If You Have Had Weight Loss Surgery.

"No man is lonely eating spaghetti; it requires so much attention." – Christopher Morley

To-Do's		Long-Term Goals

✔

✔

✔

✔

✔

✔

✔

✔

✔

✔

Do you find yourself searching for the next bite of food while you're still chewing? A lot of us eat like we're in a contest to see who can finish first, eat the most, and enjoy it the least. The simple act of slowing down and chewing your food thoroughly can prolong all of the enjoyable aspects of eating—sitting at a table with friends and family, savoring the taste, paying attention to just how amazing food can be, etc. And rushing through it can rob you of a great deal of pleasure.

Not to mention that it can also cause indigestion, increase the *amount* of food you eat, which matters if you're trying to lose weight or control your portion sizes, and ingrain yet another bad habit.

If you race through your food, you're probably just a person who thinks you are in more of a hurry than you actually need to be. Just think about it. If you're a fast eater, just ask yourself why? The answer will never be, *"Oh, I eat so fast because I'm present."* **If you're already searching your plate for what to eat next, you're already in the future.**

Commitment: At your next three meals, chew your food twice as long as you think you usually do. Try to really taste it and see if you notice anything different. See how long your meal times are. Pay attention to whether there is anything enjoyable about slowing down a meal.

☐ ☐ ☐ ☐ ☐ ☐ ☐ ☐ ☐

Journal...

_____
_____
_____
_____
_____
_____
_____
_____
_____
_____
_____
_____
_____
_____
_____
_____
_____

Enjoy The Silence

"Silence is the sleep that nourishes wisdom." – Francis Bacon

To-Do's
✔
✔
✔
✔
✔
✔
✔
✔
✔

How often is there legitimate silence in your life? "When I'm asleep," doesn't count. I mean, how often do you actually get to sit somewhere where there is no noise, very little movement, and the only sounds are the ones that you or Mother Nature are making. Probably not very often, if you're like most of us.

Modern life is busy, and busyness generally equals noise. The greater the racket, the greater our inability to focus, think, and relax. The sad thing is, you can get used to anything, including the noise. A lack of silence doesn't necessarily mean that you're not productive, happy, etc. But maybe things could be even better? **I don't know a happy person who would turn down more happiness.**

Make time for silence. Your tolerance for it will teach you something about what you're used to, and what your nervous system expects from your days.

Commitment: Start with 30 minutes of silence. Simply turn off the TV by skipping one 30-minute show. Build these quiet moments into your days as often as you can. If it recharges you, increase the time.

Long-Term Goals
☐
☐
☐
☐
☐
☐
☐
☐
☐

Journal...

Drink Red Wine

"Sorrow can be alleviated by good sleep, a bath, and a glass of wine." – Thomas Aquinas

To-Do's		Long-Term Goals

There are few self-soothing devices that are quite as effective as a simple glass of wine. When you want to feel a little different, a little switched off, it can be comforting (and devastating, if you venture into addiction) to know that relief can be as close as a glass.

But red wine has health benefits. Web MD has suggested that red wine can lead to a healthier heart, may prevent certain forms of cancer, and can help mitigate the effects of bad cholesterol (*Web MD: Health Benefits of Wine*). This, of course, can be abused. "Red wine is good for you!" could become the rallying cry of many an excuse-making, unrepentant alcoholic. "Look how healthy my heart is getting after the second bottle!"

We all know better. But the data is persuasive. Red wine, in moderation, may in fact do a body good.

Commitment: Don't avoid red wine just because you're positive that it's unhealthy. Take a wine tasting class to learn more.

Journal...

Recognize When You're Burning Out

"Burnout is nature's way of telling you, you've been going through the motions after your soul has departed; you're a zombie, a member of the walking dead, a sleepwalker." – Sam Keen

To-Do's
✔
✔
✔
✔
✔
✔
✔
✔
✔

One of the most common symptoms of depression sounds a lot like one of the most common descriptions of burnout: "An inability to enjoy things that used to give you pleasure." You can burn out on a job, a relationship, a friend, on an exercise program, or just on life itself.

And the scary part is, this happens by degrees, which is what makes it insidious. **You can reach the point of burnout and beyond without even realizing it.** You don't suddenly feel helpless, dissatisfied, lethargic, and just plain *done*. It sneaks up on you in a series of small accumulations. Physician burnout is a major problem in today's healthcare.

You have to learn how to pay attention to your energy. Your joy. Your daily pleasures. If you feel them slipping away, if you feel like things are constricting around you but you aren't sure why, ask yourself some hard questions. If you're burning out, what is causing it?

Commitment: Pay attention to the possibility of burnout. Change what you can change. Don't let it sneak up on you. Take a mini-vacation weekend getaway.

Long-Term Goals
☐
☐
☐
☐
☐
☐
☐
☐
☐

Journal...

_____
_____
_____
_____
_____
_____
_____
_____
_____
_____
_____
_____
_____
_____
_____
_____
_____
_____
_____
_____

Listen To, But Do Not Feel The Need To Act On Advice

"Parents can only give good advice or put them on the right paths, but the final forming of a person's character lies in their own hands." – Anne Frank

To-Do's

- ✔
- ✔
- ✔
- ✔
- ✔
- ✔
- ✔
- ✔
- ✔

Visit the bookstore and behold the self-help section. It threatens to buckle under the weight of all the new volumes each year. And these books proclaim to know *exactly* what you should be doing to be happier, smile more, eat less, improve self-confidence, sleep better, and so on.

Not to mention that your parents, friends, siblings, co-workers, bosses, partners, and everyone else knows how you should live. Ask them, they'll probably tell you.

The truth is, only you live your life. You can't turn your decisions, thoughts, opinions, or their results over to anyone else. Good advice can be invaluable. Few things help with perspective than listening to others. But you must listen to it openly and honestly, and then choose for yourself. Ultimately, there is no one else to blame for our mistakes, and no one else gets to take credit for our successes.

Commitment: Do not act on the advice of others simply because the advice comes from someone you trust. Think, think, think, before you act. Know what *your* opinions actually are.

Long-Term Goals

- ☐
- ☐
- ☐
- ☐
- ☐
- ☐
- ☐
- ☐
- ☐

Journal...

_____
_____
_____
_____
_____
_____
_____
_____
_____
_____
_____
_____
_____
_____
_____
_____
_____
_____
_____
_____

Take Time Off From The Gym

"You never walk out of the gym and say, 'I shouldn't have gone.'" – Taylor Kitsch

To-Do's		Long-Term Goals

Nothing will help you stick with an exercise program like choosing a program that you enjoy. Or a sport, or martial art. Point being, you will stick with the things that you like. But overzealousness can creep into anything, no matter how pleasurable or exciting it is.

Even if you're sleeping enough, refueling with proper nutrition, and working out and making good progress, it can still catch up with you. Sometimes you might start to dread going to the gym, even when things are going well. When you lose the hunger to exercise, a short break can be just what you need.

A week off can work wonders to revitalize you. During that time, you can even switch to a different, low-key form of exercise, you don't have to lay around the whole time.

Commitment: If you suddenly find that you can't look forward to exercise, take a week off. Chances are, you 'll be chomping at the bit by the time the next week rolls around. During the break, try a different leisurely activity.

Journal...

Take Control Of Your Finances

"There is a gigantic difference between earning a great deal of money and being rich." – Marlene Dietrich

To-Do's

- ✔
- ✔
- ✔
- ✔
- ✔
- ✔
- ✔
- ✔
- ✔

There are a lot of ways to remain child-like, and many of them can bring you peace and joy in your adult years. But having childish spending habits and maintaining financial ignorance are not among them. **There aren't many ways to give yourself more stress and to suck the joy out of life than in mismanaging your money.**

At the very least, you have to know what's going on with your finances. Know how much you make. Know how much your insurance costs. Know when your bills are due. Pay them on time. Avoid debt when you can, and keep track of what you owe. Don't let the hole get deeper. File your taxes. It's not how much you earn, it's how much you keep.

Once you're out of the nest, you realize that money has the power to change your life in ways that you never understood, for better or worse.

Commitment: Know how much you spend, how much you make, start saving, and work on your debt. Read a book on how to make more money. Get a secondary income stream. Even if someone else manages your finances, get a handle on it so that you could take over if you needed to.

Long-Term Goals

- ☐
- ☐
- ☐
- ☐
- ☐
- ☐
- ☐
- ☐
- ☐

Journal...

Do Something While You Watch TV

"All television is educational television. The question is: what is it teaching?" – Nicholas Johnson

To-Do's		Long-Term Goals

To-Do's

- ✔
- ✔
- ✔
- ✔
- ✔
- ✔
- ✔
- ✔

Long-Term Goals

- ☐
- ☐
- ☐
- ☐
- ☐
- ☐
- ☐
- ☐

Now, this isn't an order to start watching TV. If you can do without it, there might not be any reason to take up the habit. But you're probably someone who enjoys watching a few shows, or movies. Multitasking has its downsides, but there are ways to improve your life while engaging in the relatively passive activity of watching television.

Want to learn how to knit? You can do it while you're watching TV. Want to practice guitar scales? Ditto. Trying to sneak in a few sets of pushups, or yoga poses, or any other fitness activity you can do with your bodyweight? You can still do them with the TV on.

It's best to focus on one activity at a time, *if* the activity requires focus and concentration. Not all shows demand this. So TV is one area where you can get a little more bang for your buck, enjoying yourself and decompressing while also improving a skill.

Commitment: Find a new skill you can learn while a TV program is on.

Journal...

_____
_____
_____
_____
_____
_____
_____
_____
_____
_____
_____
_____
_____
_____
_____
_____
_____
_____
_____
_____
_____
_____

Get a Workout Partner

"Accountability breeds response-ability." – Stephen R. Covey

To-Do's		Long-Term Goals

One of the major reasons people quit—or don't even start—on their exercise routines and resolutions, is lack of accountability. We know that it's easier to break promises to ourselves than to others. It's not like skipping a workout is breaking an official contract or not doing your job. **You're only letting yourself down.**

Unless, of course, you have a workout partner. Some people love to go to the gym alone, and those are usually the people who don't have any problem motivating themselves to go. For everyone else, a partner—the right partner, who doesn't make excuses or let you make excuses either—can be just the thing to make sure you stick with it.

You want someone whose company you enjoy, but who is serious about the progress you'll make together. A partner provides motivation, help with exercises, and support.

Commitment: If you think you'd do better going to the gym, if you had a partner, get one. Start by asking someone you know who has a regular gym habit or possesses the physique you desire.

Journal...

Warn Up Properly

"I don't think that you can fake warmth. You can fake lust, jealousy, anger; those are all quite easy. But actual, genuine warmth? I don't think you can fake it." – Keira Knightley

To-Do's		Long-Term Goals
✔	With each passing year, warming up properly before exercise gets more important, particularly if you like to work out early in the day. If you're stiff and your joints are snapping, crackling, and popping, it's not yet time to jump into an intense workout.	☐
✔		☐
✔	It's also possible to *overdo* a warmup and expend way too much time and energy on it. **We literally just want to get your body warm.** You can put your heater on while driving to the gym, then spend five minutes on the treadmill, and maybe you're good to go. But get a light sweat going.	☐
✔		☐
✔	It is also possible to warm up with a lighter, specific version of the exercise you're about to do. So if you're working up to a heavy bench press, you can start by bench pressing the bar, then 95 lbs, and on up in increments. This will warm up the specific joints and muscles that you'll be using.	☐
✔		☐
✔		☐
✔	**Commitment:** Start warming up properly, but don't overdo it. Light stretches and jumping jacks are easy ideas.	☐

Journal...

_____
_____
_____
_____
_____
_____
_____
_____
_____
_____
_____
_____
_____
_____
_____
_____
_____
_____
_____
_____
_____
_____

Try Interval Training

"You will always reap greater rewards by exercising at the more intense side of the spectrum." – James Driver

To-Do's

- ✔
- ✔
- ✔
- ✔
- ✔
- ✔
- ✔
- ✔

Long-Term Goals

- ☐
- ☐
- ☐
- ☐
- ☐
- ☐
- ☐
- ☐

Anything that gets your heart rate up has a fat-burning effect. And, while you might be one of the cardio nuts who loves to zone out for 45 minutes on a treadmill, there are ways to get the benefits of cardio in substantially less time. **And we all need to learn how to maximize our time.**

High Intensity Interval Training—HIIT—refers to a brief period of intense exercise (the interval), followed by a reduction in effort, before starting again. For instance, you might sprint for 100 yards and then walk for 20 yards, before beginning to sprint again. Or jumping rope for one minute and then walking in place for 20 seconds. You get the idea.

The intensity puts your fat burners on full blast, and will save you time in the long run. You might be able to jog for 45 minutes, but nobody sprints for that long. If a few sprints would save you time and get you even better results, it might be an experiment worth trying.

Commitment: On what you would call a "cardio day," try HIIT instead.

Journal...

_____
_____
_____
_____
_____
_____
_____
_____
_____
_____
_____
_____
_____
_____
_____
_____
_____
_____
_____
_____
_____
_____
_____

Try Tabata Workouts

"That which does not kill us, make us stronger." – Friedrich Nietzsche

To-Do's		Long-Term Goals

Tabata is a specific variant of the High Intensity Interval, and it's an absolute killer. But there may not be a better high intensity workout **for those who can handle it.** And it only takes four minutes, so there's little chance that you'll find a shorter workout. But it's going to be a long four minutes.

The protocol is simple. You choose an exercise that you can go all-out on for 20 seconds. Then you rest for 10 seconds. That's one round. You do eight rounds like this and you're done. Good exercises for Tabata are kettlebell swings, sprints, rowing on a machine, push ups, or the squat variation of your choice. Hire a trainer to help you.

To do Tabata correctly, you'll need a timer. When you only get 10 seconds of rest, it's easy to take a couple more. And when you know you have to go hard for 20 seconds, you don't want to look down at a stopwatch and lose a couple seconds' worth of effort.

Commitment: Tabata can be a useful part of an exercise routine, but it's not for everyone. Give it a try and mix it into your schedule every week if you like the results and the time you save.

Journal...

Lift At Different Tempos

"Instead of thinking that's a nice tune, you start thinking is it the right pace, is it the right tempo? That is the death knell for artists." – Alison Moyet

To-Do's		Long-Term Goals
✔		☐
✔		☐
✔		☐
✔		☐
✔		☐
✔		☐
✔		☐
✔		☐
✔		☐

It is possible to overcomplicate the act of lifting weights. At its most simple, each exercise has a point A and a point B, and performing the exercise just means moving between the two points enough times to get the result you want. But one thing nobody talks about much is lifting tempo.

Sometimes, particularly if you have a nagging pain in a joint or muscle, lifting quickly can make the pain worse, or at least, impossible to ignore, while slowing down and taking 3-4 seconds to execute the rep might feel painless. **Speed at the end ranges of motion is one of the most frequent causes of weight room injuries.**

First and foremost, find the tempo that is pain-free. This will vary at different times in your life. But experiment with slow tempos, even at speeds that feel exaggeratedly slow. Some bodybuilders swear by it. Others think that it's nonsense. Give yourself a chance to decide for yourself.

Commitment: During your next workout, lift weights slower than you usually do. Add a couple of seconds to each rep, and *count* so you actually know you're doing it. Note your results and sensations in your training log.

Journal...

Upgrade Your Wardrobe

"Clothes are fun. The designers have so much fun making them, you should have fun wearing them, too." – Rita Ora

To-Do's		Long-Term Goals

When people get depressed, one of the first things they stop paying attention to is how they look. It's not uncommon to see a depressed man who has suddenly gone for a week without shaving, or a woman who has not done her hair in just as long. It just doesn't seem to be worth the effort, when there's no point to anything.

But there can be a point to maintaining and taking pride in your wardrobe, even if you've never experienced depression. When you know you look good and are dressed well, it's hard not to feel more confident. Taking the energy to make sure your clothes are washed, ironed, new enough to not look shabby, and that they fit you well, is not the behavior of a fussy diva. You don't have to be a narcissist to want to look your best.

This applies even more so if you've had weight loss surgery.

Commitment: Start paying more attention to your wardrobe. Replace anything that is old or faded. Take pride in your appearance.

Journal...

Recycle

"If you want grown-ups to recycle, just tell their kids the importance of recycling, and they'll be all over it." – Bill Nye

To-Do's

- ✔
- ✔
- ✔
- ✔
- ✔
- ✔
- ✔

Long-Term Goals

- ☐
- ☐
- ☐
- ☐
- ☐
- ☐
- ☐

One day the universe is going to wind down and the party will go on without us. But while we're here, there are things we can do to ensure that this is a world worth living in, and that it will remain so for our children, and their children, and on down the line. **It is our duty to leave this planet thriving for the generations to come.**

One of the easiest things that everyone can do is to recycle whatever they can. This does not mean going full-bore Obsessive Compulsive Disorder. It can be as simple as getting a recycling bin and dividing the trash from the recyclables when you have something to put in a bin. You'll be surprised, once you start paying attention, at how much more infrequently you have to put trash bins out.

Commitment: Get a recycling bin. Learn what you can recycle and do it. The planet will thank you. Your great grandchildren will thank you.

Journal...

_____
_____
_____
_____
_____
_____
_____
_____
_____
_____
_____
_____
_____
_____
_____
_____
_____
_____
_____
_____
_____
_____
_____
_____

Start A Book Club

"A classic is a book that doesn't have to be written again." – W.E.B. Dubois

To-Do's		Long-Term Goals

✔

✔

✔

✔

✔

✔

✔

It can be hard to make time to read, even if you love it. As with so many things, accountability can be key. If you don't read, unless you're an English student or professor, no one is likely to notice or worry about it. A book club can be the accountability you need.

One of the best things about a book club is that you'll actually talk about the ideas in the book, and hear perspectives that you wouldn't have thought of. It's always fun to get together with friends, but **there are few things as stimulating as a group of people who like each other, exchanging ideas and engaging in respectful debate.**

Better yet, if each person in the group takes a turn picking a book, you'll probably wind up reading books you never would have heard of.

Commitment: Start a book club (or join one). You can also use audio books to help ease the process.

☐ ☐ ☐ ☐ ☐ ☐ ☐

Journal...

Sleep In A Dark Room

"The amount of sleep required by the average person is five minutes more." – Wilson Mizener

To-Do's

- ✔
- ✔
- ✔
- ✔
- ✔
- ✔

Long-Term Goals

- ☐
- ☐
- ☐
- ☐
- ☐
- ☐

Unless you sleep in a cave, the room you sleep in could probably be a little darker. Or maybe a lot darker. You have more control over your sleeping environment when you're at home, but ideally you can replicate ideal sleeping conditions wherever you are.

One of the easiest ways to cut down on the amount of light in the room while you sleep is to get a sleep mask. For $10 you can cover your eyes with a mask and get a better chance at sleep.

There are also special blackout curtains that are nearly impenetrable to light. Putting a blanket or towel over the cracks under doors and around windows can also help. Also, don't let the light from a television disturb your sleep.

Commitment: Sleep in as dark a room as possible. Remove the television set from the bedroom.

Journal...

Track Calories Over A Week Not A Day

"Don't compare yourself with someone else's version of happy or thin. Accepting yourself burns the most calories." – Caroline Rhea

To-Do's		Long-Term Goals

Counting calories gets a bad rap, and it can certainly be taken too far. But the truth is that fat/weight loss is simple. Not all calories are created equal, but losing weight means taking in fewer calories than you expend, and gaining weight means consuming more calories than you expend. **Of course being healthy is more complicated than that, but think of calorie counting as the start line.**

We've already talked about keeping a food journal. I'd like to suggest a variant of calorie counting. If you find daily caloric planning too cumbersome, consider instead that you can track calories across an entire week. You can still evaluate your results. If they're satisfactory, it can be a lot easier to say "I'm going to take in 1000 fewer calories this week," than to try to break that up into seven daily increments. That's only 142 Cal a day, or just not having the muffin for breakfast or skipping the cream in your coffee. This equals approximately a 15-pound weight loss in one year, and who wouldn't want that?

Setting a finish line is a different task, but you need a start line in order to have a journey.

Commitment: Try counting and adjusting your calories over a week, instead of each day. Make small changes. If it works for you this could free up a lot of headspace and planning.

Journal...

Wash Your Linens

"I really like doing the laundry, because I succeed at it. But I loathe putting it away. It is already clean." – Jenny Holzer

To-Do's

- ✓
- ✓
- ✓
- ✓
- ✓
- ✓
- ✓

Long-Term Goals

- ☐
- ☐
- ☐
- ☐
- ☐
- ☐
- ☐

Even if you do laundry every day, it can be easy to forget to wash your linens and bedding. But think about the germ traps your sheets can be. Even if you shower right before you get in bed, you're still sloughing off skin and hair during the night. Say you wash your linens every week. That's seven days' worth of gunk, even if you can't see it. **Sometimes it's the stuff we can't see that gets us.**

To say nothing of the dust mites that live on our mattresses. When sheets get swirled around in the night, or they drag across the ground while you're making your bed, they can pick up so much crud. This doesn't even count the pet lovers out there who let their animals sleep on the bed.

And again, even if you can't see it, you know your bedding could be cleaner. You know it.

Commitment: Wash your bedding at least once a week.

Journal...

Get A Lint Roller

"Juliet's version of cleanliness was next to godliness, which was to say it was erratic, past all understanding and was seldom seen." – Terry Pratchett

To-Do's		Long-Term Goals

✔

✔

✔

✔

✔

✔

✔

No matter how well you clean and iron your clothes, and even if your tailor is a magician and your wardrobe couldn't fit better, the effect can get lost quickly if you strut your stuff while covered in lint, hair, dog hair, etc. If you have a pet, you know exactly what this means. But even if you don't, hair and lint can accumulate on clothes.

A couple of passes with a lint roller can take care of this. It's basically a roll of tape on a handle. You run it over your clothes and voila, you're no longer covered in hair. The kind of things most likely to be picked up with a roller are often most visible against black clothing, so keep that in mind.

Looking good leads to feeling good. But it's often the small details that will make or break your day.

Commitment: Get a lint roller. Get in the habit of checking your pants and your front to see if you need it before going out.

☐ ☐ ☐ ☐ ☐ ☐ ☐

Journal...

_____
_____
_____
_____
_____
_____
_____
_____
_____
_____
_____
_____
_____
_____
_____
_____
_____
_____
_____
_____
_____
_____

Never Drive Drunk

"Friends never let friends drive drunk." – Drunk Driving Prevention Campaign

To-Do's		Long-Term Goals

In 2014, 9,967 people died in drunk driving crashes. This does not get into the amount of injuries caused or dollars spent in DUI related accidents. In 2013, 28.7 million Americans admitted to driving under the influence of alcohol (www.madd.org.)

If you have had anything to drink, don't drive. **There are no justifications for blood alcohol limits and "being able to handle it."** Especially now with easy and quick on-demand car services such as Uber or Lift.

If you've had anything to drink, do not get behind the wheel. Ever. It's not worth ruining anyone's life over, including your own.

Commitment: Never drink and drive. Ever. Download the Uber or Lift app and start using them. I do.

Journal...

Find A Friend

"Remember that the most valuable antiques are dear old friends." – H. Jackson Brown, Jr.

To-Do's

- ✔
- ✔
- ✔
- ✔
- ✔
- ✔
- ✔
- ✔

Many of our childhoods revolved around our friends. Want to come play? When will we see each other again? What do you want to do tonight? Who's your homeroom teacher? What should we go do? We'd talk to each other, listen to each other, and just bask in the fact that someone else also struggled on the math test. We felt understood.

It's strange that close friendships are often rare in adult life. **No one ever stops needing to feel understood.** No one ever stops needing a sympathetic ear or a pep talk when things are hard. No one wakes up one day and says, "Guess that's it. I finally know that I'll never want to sit around and laugh with a friend again."

Nothing as mundane as "being busy" is a good excuse for not nurturing friendships. And now with social media and texting, it's never been as easy to reach out and make friends.

Commitment: Get back in touch with an old friend this week. If that's not an option, reach out and make a new friend.

Long-Term Goals

- ☐
- ☐
- ☐
- ☐
- ☐
- ☐
- ☐
- ☐

Journal...

Ditch The Soda

"Diet cola is my absolute favorite drink in the world; I used to drink four cans a day. But to help me cut down, I've turned it into a treat. Now, instead of having dessert, I'll have a can of diet soda. Putting a limit on how often I can drink it has helped me appreciate it more." – Kaley Cuoco

To-Do's		Long-Term Goals

Soda, diet or otherwise, is never going to be the healthiest thing in the world. But neither is it the boogeyman some people have tried to turn it into, despite it having practically zero nutritional value. **The key, as with everything, is to understand what you are putting into your body when you drink soda.**

It's easy to become dependent on caffeine, which explains a lot of people's reliance on soda. Not everyone likes coffee or tea. But there is also the feel of the carbonation, the taste—we can become addicted to the habit and feeling of soda apart from the caffeine. And of course, not every soda is caffeinated.

If you have a soda habit, you're not enjoying it as much as you could. If you don't want to cut it out entirely, at least limit it so that you'll appreciate it more when you get it.

Commitment: If you're a soda drinker, reduce your intake by fifty percent this week. Pay attention to how your body responds. Notice if the swelling in your ankles decrease or if the pain in your joints get better.

Journal...

Practice Daily Affirmations

"To give someone a blessing is the most significant affirmation we can offer." – Henri Nouwen

To-Do's

✔

✔

✔

✔

✔

✔

✔

✔

Long-Term Goals

☐ ☐ ☐ ☐ ☐ ☐ ☐ ☐ ☐

This tip comes with a qualifier: there are people who simply find the idea of daily affirmations to be too cheesy and fail to give it an honest try. If that's you, don't feel the need to try. But be open to the fact that not every affirmation needs to have you smiling at yourself in the mirror, parroting something cheery like, "I'm active, I'm attractive, I'm in demand!" That probably would make most peoples' eyes roll.

There is power to the "fake it until you make it" or "Smile until you feel like smiling" mindset. As you come up with affirmations for yourself that you can reinforce through repetition, just make a short list of things you like about yourself. That's it.

"I'm kind." "I'm generous." "I'm an amazing guitarist." "I'm honest." "I'm a good parent." "I'm a hard worker." Even if you already know these things, repeating them to yourself, at the very least, will replace the negative things you might be saying to yourself in the absence of affirmations.

Commitment: Make a list of one dozen affirmations that don't make you roll your eyes. Say them to yourself each day this week at the beginning of your day.

Journal...

_____
_____
_____
_____
_____
_____
_____
_____
_____
_____
_____
_____
_____
_____
_____
_____
_____
_____
_____

Celebrate Your Successes

"The celebration...you cannot practice it or anything. It's a moment when the excitement of your goal make you react to the moment." – Peter Bondra

To-Do's

- ✔
- ✔
- ✔
- ✔
- ✔
- ✔
- ✔

Long-Term Goals

- ☐
- ☐
- ☐
- ☐
- ☐
- ☐
- ☐

All progress is worth celebrating. This can be easy to forget if you only measure progress and success against the achievements of others, especially after weight loss surgery. **But we always have the chance to be better than we were yesterday.**

Every step you take towards a goal is worth celebrating. Every time you make the right choice, or gain ground in a battle you're fighting against your bad habits, it's worth celebrating. All progress should be acknowledged and celebrated. This doesn't mean you need to have a parade because you're finally brushing your teeth every day, but find a way to make yourself feel good, formally, about your progress.

Commitment: Take an inventory of the goals you're pursuing. Track the progress you're making. Do something nice for yourself regularly, just to tell yourself that you're proud of how well you're doing.

Journal...

_____

June

Don't Compare Yourself To Others

"You can be the moon and still be jealous of the stars." – Gary Allan

To-Do's		Long-Term Goals

✔

✔

✔

✔

✔

✔

✔

✔

✔

✔

This tip is easier said than done. You can't really snap your fingers at a shy person and say, "Hey, be less shy!" and expect it to work. Neither can you snap your fingers at yourself, order yourself to stop making these comparisons, and expect it to work.

It takes time and effort. But the thing you *can* do right now is to acknowledge that there is no point in comparing yourself to someone else. **You are *not* someone else.** Maybe you can get what they have, or achieve the same success, but if you are wishing you were more like them, you don't have it yet. So acknowledge how you feel, but then, if it's really important to you to become more like the person you're comparing yourself to, you have to come up with a plan.

When you're thinking about something as arbitrary as physical attractiveness, natural talent, etc., there may not be a path to the things you desire. Acknowledge this and focus on what you can control.

Commitment: The next time you find yourself comparing yourself unfavorably to someone, pay attention and ask yourself why you're doing it. Remember, in the history of time, before you were born, there's never been anyone like you. And after you die, there will never be another person just like you.

☐ ☐ ☐ ☐ ☐ ☐ ☐ ☐ ☐ ☐

Journal...

Be Inspired, Not Intimidated

"Intimidation doesn't last very long." – Lenny Wilkens

To-Do's		Long-Term Goals
✔	Let's use an example from the fitness world. Say you want to bench press 500 pounds. It's a lofty, long-term goal, but you're committed, even though you're currently benching 95 pounds. So you soldier on, and then one day you go to the gym and you see someone actually benching 500 pounds. You can't believe how much weight it is. The bar is actually bending!	☐

Let's use an example from the fitness world. Say you want to bench press 500 pounds. It's a lofty, long-term goal, but you're committed, even though you're currently benching 95 pounds. So you soldier on, and then one day you go to the gym and you see someone actually benching 500 pounds. You can't believe how much weight it is. The bar is actually bending!

Here's the moment where you choose. You set a big, audacious goal, and you were committed. Now that you see what it actually means, up close and personal, you get to decide whether you are now intimidated or inspired. **Inspiration is always the right choice.**

There will always be someone bigger, smaller, smarter, taller, sexier, more well-read, more educated, faster, younger, and so on. You can only control what you can control. Work on you. Take inspiration from everyone who is making progress. Do not let their progress intimidate you and make you second guess the value of your own goals.

Commitment: Whenever you are intimidated by someone else's progress, tell yourself that you are inspired instead. Then take that motivation to help you work even harder. Set a newer, even more audacious goal.

Journal...

Test Yourself

"Accept the challenges so that you can feel the exhilaration of victory." – George S. Patton

To-Do's
✔
✔
✔
✔
✔
✔

There are a lot of ways to set challenges for yourself in your fitness, and periodic tests of endurance or strength can be a fun way to see just how far you've come in your program.

For instance, if you run a mile every day at a leisurely pace, why not take a day to see just how fast you can run the mile? Or take a day to run two miles? If you go into the gym and do three sets of ten reps on the squat every day, why not go in once in a while and see if you do a set of twenty? The numbers don't matter; what matters is that you test yourself. **But this applies in any area of your life, not just fitness.**

So, sooner rather than later, set up a competition against yourself. You'll win just by trying.

Commitment: Find a challenge for yourself in your preferred area of fitness.

Long-Term Goals

☐ ☐ ☐ ☐ ☐ ☐

Journal...

Walk With Weight

"Farmers walks and bear hug carries are my personal favorite moves and tend to be some of the best bang-for-the-buck choices." – Dan John

To-Do's		Long-Term Goals

We've talked a lot about "useful" strength in this book so far. One of the images that always gets brought up is that of "farm strength." You can probably picture someone slinging bales of hay, or carrying heavy bags across a farmyard. **But anyone can develop "farm strength."**

The simple act of walking with weight can work wonders for your posture, core, and reveal asymmetries in your strength.   There are three varieties we'll talk about. Walking with weight in your hands, like suitcases, walking with weight crushed against you like a bear hug, and walking while holding weight overhead.

You can do the in-hand carries with dumbbells, kettlebells, or anything else that you can hold on to. For the bear hug, I recommended getting a bag of sand and testing it out. If it's not too heavy, you can put two sandbags in a heavy duffel bag. Once you can walk comfortably, carrying and holding, with heavy weight, you'll be amazed at how much easier some of your other lifts will begin to feel.

Commitment: Add loaded carries to your workout once per week.

Journal…

Shave Your Calluses

"When I came off the boat I was very proud of the thick calluses which had developed on my feet. But now, I am struggling to get into my favorite high heels which is a shame, as I have so many." – Pamela Stephenson

To-Do's		Long-Term Goals
✓	If you put in any serious time lifting weights, you're going to develop calluses on your hands. And if you're a walker or runner, they'll eventually start trying to take over your feet.	☐
✓	Lifting gloves seem like an easy solution, but I'd like to recommend against them. If you're wearing gloves to prevent callus build up, there's a better way. Gloves	☐
✓	prevent you from being as in touch with the weights as possible. **The more you can feel, the better aware you'll be if a weight shifts in your hand.**	☐
✓		☐
✓	Also, once you're lifting heavy, if you have a layer of calluses at the top of your palm, a barbell or dumbbell can cause them to bunch up and tear. This can be a setback if	☐
✓	you have to take time off from lifting to let your hand mend itself.	☐
✓	Get a shaver. It's not glamorous but if you use it every time you're in the shower, you'll never have this issue again.	☐
✓	**Commitment:** Buy a callus shaver. The Ped Egg is inexpensive and easy to use.	☐

Journal...

_____
_____
_____
_____
_____
_____
_____
_____
_____
_____
_____
_____
_____
_____
_____
_____
_____
_____
_____
_____

Don't Play Devil's Advocate All The Time

"People have confused playing devil's advocate with being intelligent." – Cecily Strong

To-Do's
✔
✔
✔
✔
✔
✔
✔

There's nothing wrong with someone in a conversation being willing to argue and object to sloppy thinking, or to ask for clarification of a point, even if it can come off as combative. But it's really tedious to have someone around who thinks **serial contrarianism** is a religion.

There are times when playing Devil's Advocate is useful. There are times when it's beyond obnoxious. This usually happens when someone has assumed that their duty is to question everything. This comes in the guise of free-thinking, often by someone who is willing to talk the loudest. But it's usually from someone who has not done their homework.

Question what you need to question. Don't be a jerk about it. Contribute when you can. Lift others up if possible.

Commitment: Take a break from playing Devil's Advocate for a week.

Long-Term Goals
☐
☐
☐
☐
☐
☐
☐

Journal...

Take A Boxing Class

"A computer once beat me at chess, but it was no match for me at kickboxing." – Emo Philips, comedian

To-Do's

- ✓
- ✓
- ✓
- ✓
- ✓
- ✓
- ✓

Long-Term Goals

- ☐
- ☐
- ☐
- ☐
- ☐
- ☐
- ☐

This is not a summons for you to quit your job and become a professional boxer, or Muay Thai fighter, or a wrestler, or a Jiu Jitsu fiend. But taking a boxing class—or a class centered on any other combat sport—can be a great way of mixing it up, and it's a type of cardio unlike any other.

Many first timers in a boxing class can't believe how difficult it can be just to hold your arms up for three rounds, in a fighting stance. And that's before you even start throwing punches! The footwork, particularly the lateral movement, is often unlike anything people have done, and can work wonders for mobility and coordination.

And it goes without saying, there are upsides to learning how to punch, kick, and react in certain situations.

Commitment: Sign up for a boxing class. Go into it with an open mind, just focusing on the workout you get. Afterwards, sign up to go again before you can change your mind.

Journal...

Write Yourself A Letter From The Future

"I would have answered your letter sooner, but you didn't send one." –Goodman Ace

To-Do's
✔
✔
✔
✔
✔

If you could write to yourself, 30 years from now, what would you want the present-day version of yourself to know? Are there things right now that are taking up too much headspace and energy, that you would tell yourself to get over? Would you remind yourself to stay close to your family? To save more money? To get back in touch with someone you had lost track of?

It doesn't have to be a hyper-introspective exercise either, you can just try to make yourself laugh. Tell yourself about how great the future is, and how things have changed.

Commitment: Write yourself a letter from 5, 10, 20, 50 years into the future.

Long-Term Goals
☐
☐
☐
☐
☐

Journal...

Avoid Cruelty

"Cruelty is a misuse of pain." – Annie Dillard

To-Do's

- ✔
- ✔
- ✔
- ✔
- ✔
- ✔
- ✔

Pain can be a wonderful teacher, if it changes your behavior. When something hurts, if you reflect, you will always be able to say, "This is where it went wrong," or "That's what I should have avoided." Pain is a signal, and it arrives because sometimes things are just going to hurt.

Cruelty is different. Cruelty, whether we are receiving or practicing it, is pain *with intention.* **Cruelty is never an accident.** Its only goal is to wound. Therefore, there can't be anything productive about it, and the only lesson to be learned is that sometimes people can be cruel. That's it.

If you are cruel, you may become unforgettable to someone in the worst way. If you've ever experienced cruelty from someone, you know this can be true. There's just no reason for it, ever.

Commitment: Do not be cruel. Wayne Dyer said, "Whenever given the choice between being kind and being right, choose kind." Always choose kind.

Long-Term Goals

- ☐
- ☐
- ☐
- ☐
- ☐
- ☐
- ☐

Journal...

Keep A Dream Journal

"You have to dream before your dreams can come true." – A. P. J. Abdul Kalam

To-Do's
✔
✔
✔
✔
✔
✔

The world of dreams is the world of the subconscious trying to unpack itself at the end of the day. We don't always remember our dreams, but we probably do forget most of them if we don't write them down. Keeping a dream journal can be a fascinating exercise in self-observation.

What do your dreams say about you? Writing them down, as often as you're able to retain them after waking, will help you spot patterns and changes in your dreams over the long-term.

If nothing else, dream journals get very entertaining, very quickly.

Commitment: Keep a dream journal next to your bed. Upon waking, jot down anything you remember about your night's sleep.

Long-Term Goals
☐
☐
☐
☐
☐
☐

Journal...

Walk To The Restaurant

"I never eat in a restaurant that's over a hundred feet off the ground and won't stand still." – Calvin Trillin

To-Do's
✔
✔
✔
✔
✔

Long-Term Goals
☐
☐
☐
☐
☐

Eating out can be one of life's greatest pleasures. Someone else prepares your food, and all you have to do is sit there, smack your lips, and revel in it. But eating out often, depending on what you order, can be a recipe for weight gain. When we eat out, we tend to choose our favorite things. If our favorite things aren't healthy...well, you see what I'm getting at.

However, there is one easy way to defray *some* of the fitness cost of indulging in a decadent meal at a restaurant—walk. If it's within walking distance, walk to the restaurant, and walk home.

Commitment: Walk to the restaurant, eat smart, and walk back.

Journal...

Stop Complaining

"People won't have time for you if you are always angry or complaining." – Stephen Hawking

To-Do's		Long-Term Goals
✔	Let's make a distinction between venting and complaining. Venting is blowing off steam. You just get it all out with a sympathetic ear and then you feel better when it's done. Then you move on. It's a way to bark and complain a *little* as a means of feeling better afterwards.	☐
✔		☐
✔	But complaining never makes anyone feel better, unless complaining has become the primary source of pleasure, and how sad is that to think about? We all know someone who complains because...well, because that's what they do.	☐
✔		☐
✔	Don't be that person. Vent when you need to. Avoid the complaining habit like the plague.	☐
✔	**Commitment:** The next time you say something negative, ask yourself if you're complaining or venting. If you feel worse afterwards, it's probably complaining. If you continue to talk about it, then you are definitely complaining.	☐
✔		☐

Journal...

_____
_____
_____
_____
_____
_____
_____
_____
_____
_____
_____
_____
_____
_____
_____
_____
_____
_____
_____
_____
_____
_____
_____

Define Fame

"So, my happiness doesn't come from money or fame. My happiness comes from seeing life without struggle." –
Nicky Minaj

To-Do's		Long-Term Goals
✔		☐
✔		☐
✔		☐
✔		☐
✔		☐
✔		☐
✔		☐
✔		☐

With the rise of social media and reality TV, it's never been easier to become "famous." That's only meant to be slightly tongue in cheek. Everyone has a way to broadcast their voice now, even when (especially when?) we don't seem to have much to say.

There's nothing wrong with wanting to reach people, or help people, or make people laugh. But when we have the urge to post something on Facebook or Twitter, it can be enlightening to stop and ask ourselves why we're doing it. Chances are, it's about building our own fame.

"I want to be famous." Think about what this means. It is literally saying, "It is important to me that as many people as possible are simply *aware of me."* What could be a sadder, or more hollow, goal? If increased fame makes us more useful, then it's worth pursuing. **Fame as *the* goal is empty.**

Commitment: If you want to be famous, ask yourself why. Will your fame serve a greater purpose? If so, what is that purpose?

Journal...

Think Of Strength As a Skill

"Strength does not come from physical capacity. It comes from an indomitable will." – Mahatma Gandhi

To-Do's		Long-Term Goals

You don't have to work out until you're purple in the face and collapsing on the floor in order to know that you got something out of it. Neither do you need to seek out sore muscles as proof that you're working hard. If your goal is to get stronger, consider that strength is a skill.

If you do this, you can start to see your workouts as practice sessions. You aren't looking for the sensations of a hard workout, **you're looking at progress and practice.** It can also relieve you of notions of the amount of time you "should" be spending at the gym.

If you focus on strength—not that everyone should, this tip is for those who prioritize it—then simply viewing it as results-oriented practice means you may never even think of it as exercise at all. For some people, this is what keeps them coming back.

Commitment: Find a lift that you'd like to get stronger at. Now practice it. Record your improvement in that skill.

Journal...

Make A To-Do List

"To Do Today, 1/17/08
1. Sit and think
2. Reach enlightenment
3. Feed the cats – Jared Kintz

To-Do's		Long-Term Goals
✔	It's hard not to feel better about life when you know you're getting things done. And the best way to know you're getting things done is to cross things off of a to do list. **There is a real satisfaction in crossing something off, or checking a box, and knowing that you made it happen.**	☐
✔		☐
✔	Living by the seat of the pants can have its charms, and often masquerades under the guise of "spontaneity." If you think you can remember everything you need to get done, at some point this optimism is going to catch up to you and you'll pay a price for it. Get in the habit of keeping a to do list and you'll always know what you need to get done.	☐
✔		☐
✔		☐
✔	**Commitment:** Keep a to do list of the five major tasks you need to get done for the day. Then review it at the end of the day. Mark off what you've accomplished. Move uncompleted items to the next day.	☐

Journal...

_____
_____
_____
_____
_____
_____
_____
_____
_____
_____
_____
_____
_____
_____
_____
_____
_____
_____
_____
_____
_____
_____
_____
_____

Watch A Documentary

"Doing a documentary is about discovering, being open, learning, and following curiosity." – Spike Jonze

To-Do's	
✔	
✔	
✔	
✔	
✔	
✔	

Long-Term Goals

☐
☐
☐
☐
☐
☐

Watching a TV program, or a movie, is a largely passive activity. You sit, stare, boot up the next episode. Occasionally you might think. But not many shows demand much of us. And yet, the pleasure and escapism that movies and shows can offer us is not something to shy away from.

Watching a documentary can be the best of both worlds. **The best documentaries tell a story as they teach.** They are meticulously crafted and provocative in the best ways. It is a way to learn without necessarily feeling like, "Oh, I guess it's time to sit down and learn."

Commitment: Watch a documentary with a friend. If it's on a subject that you're less familiar with, so much the better. Afterwards, discuss the film.

Journal...

_____
_____
_____
_____
_____
_____
_____
_____
_____
_____
_____
_____
_____
_____
_____
_____
_____
_____
_____
_____
_____
_____
_____
_____
_____
_____
_____

What Does It Mean To Know Something

"We get sucked into the Internet and streaming information, and it's time to just unplug and look within." –
Jonathan Cain

To-Do's
✔
✔
✔
✔
✔
✔

Knowing where to find an answer can feel like knowing the answer. Why take the trouble to learn something when you can just look it up? But something is lost in this process. There was a time when, if you couldn't figure something out, you might never get an answer.

But even if you don't succeed after grappling with a problem, there is joy to be had in the mental effort of trying to figure something out. The next time you want to know something, don't be so quick to look it up. See if you can figure it out for yourself, as long as there's no time pressure.

Commitment: The next time you want to know something, don't look it up immediately. Spend some time grappling with the question and try to enjoy the process.

Long-Term Goals
☐
☐
☐
☐
☐
☐

Journal...

Working Memory vs. Long Term Memory

"Happiness is good health and a bad memory." – Ingrid Bergman

To-Do's

- ✔
- ✔
- ✔
- ✔
- ✔
- ✔
- ✔

Long-Term Goals

- ☐
- ☐
- ☐
- ☐
- ☐
- ☐
- ☐

If you feel more distractible than usual, or your memory seems to be going bad, here's something to think about. In his book *The Shallows: What The Internet Is Doing To Our Brains,* Nicholas Carr breaks our memory down into short-term memory (or, working memory) and long-term.

He says to think of working memory as a bunch of post-it notes. And long-term memory is a filing cabinet. **Our ability to remember things is a function of how many of the post-it notes we can get into the filing cabinet.** So if you tell yourself, "I've got to do this," and you forget what you were supposed to do because then you click on five more articles, scan them, then watch a funny cat video, you've lost your post-it note on the way to the filing cabinet.

Commitment: Just think about this. If it sounds familiar, cut back on your Internet use until you feel it change. Write everything down.

Journal...

Train Your Brain

"The nice thing about doing a crossword puzzle is, you know there is a solution." – Stephen Sondheim

To-Do's		Long-Term Goals

✔

✔

✔

✔

✔

✔

✔

Your brain needs to be trained if it's going to work to its full potential. Even the most elite neurologists will tell you that we still don't really know how the brain works. And yet, it does everything that matters. **Your brain constructs your reality and allows you to function.** It's an incredible machine that we can't take for granted.

Putting your brain through its daily paces can mean something as simple as doing crosswords, playing Sudoku, or logic puzzles. If crosswords don't come naturally to you, it's because your brain isn't trained to do them. Ditto for any other puzzle game you can think of.

Brain games have been shown to prevent—or at least delay—the onset of various forms of dementia.

Commitment: Work at least one brain game per day into your schedule. This could be as simple as doing math problems in your head.

☐ ☐ ☐ ☐ ☐ ☐ ☐

Journal...

Save Money Regularly

"I'm thankful for the three ounce Ziploc bag, so that I have somewhere to put my savings." – Paula Poundstone

To-Do's		Long-Term Goals
✔		☐
✔		☐
✔		☐
✔		☐
✔		☐
✔		☐
✔		☐
✔		☐

Not many Americans have a substantive savings account. Depending on who you ask, everyone should have between six months' and a year's worth of savings in the bank, just in case we lose our jobs, get in a car wreck, have a health catastrophe, and/or any of the other rough reversals of fortune that are part of life.

It's not easy to save, psychologically, especially when it feels like we can barely make ends meet. **The key to saving regularly, like so many of the other tips in this book, is to make it a habit.** Could you save 10% of any income you make? What about 5%? 1%?

Probably. Once you learn to live without it, and you can, you can stop thinking about it, and it will keep growing without you.

Commitment: Commit to saving a certain percentage of any income you make. Set up a special "secret" bank account where money from side income are automatically deposited.

Journal...

Take The Stairs

"This morning I was laughing at my cat who was running up the stairs and slipped, and pretended like it didn't happen." – Jayma Mays

To-Do's		Long-Term Goals

How often do you have to climb? I don't mean climbing up into a tree or scaling a mountain, but the simple act of stepping up to a higher elevation? Chances are, there are always elevators available to you, or you're wearing high heels, or you don't have time to take the stairs or or or or or....

You get the picture. **Every day is made of small moments.** Each moment is made of small choices. Most of those choices get turned into habits, so we're on autopilot a lot of the time. Most of those habits probably don't turn into exercise. But this is an easy one.

If you are somewhere where you could occasionally take the stairs—your office, your apartment, that second story restaurant you like—then take the stairs as often as you can. It'll help you develop extra leg strength, it'll make your heart work a little in the best way, and most importantly, *you won't lose the ability to walk up stairs.*

Commitment: Take the stairs whenever you can.

Journal...

Order The Special

"The simplification of anything is always sensational." – Gilbert K. Chesterton

To-Do's		Long-Term Goals

✔

✔

✔

✔

✔

✔

✔

Some aspects of life are, and will, remain complex. Human emotions, aging, relationships, they're all tricky business. **But some things can be simple.** Consider the act of going to a restaurant and being presented with a dizzying array of menu options.

To paraphrase TV star RuPaul, he said (I'm paraphrasing), "When I go into a restaurant, I ask what the special is. That's what I order, and then I don't have to waste time reading a menu. Doesn't have to be harder than that."

Whether or not you apply this to your restaurant habits, you can probably see how it could apply to other arenas of life. Many, many things in life can be more simple than we make them.

Commitment: Pay attention to your activities this week, and figure out where your time goes, even if it's two minutes that disappear into the reading of a menu. Choose one activity and simplify.

☐
☐
☐
☐
☐
☐
☐

Journal...

Learn To Draw

"Life is the art of drawing without an eraser." – John W. Gardner

To-Do's		Long-Term Goals

One of the essential skills for early anatomists was the ability to draw. Because photography did not yet exist, an organ had to be sketched from as many angles as possible in order to be studied and anthologized. Just as you would not study a blurry roadmap to guide you, you would not want your surgeon to learn about the heart from poorly rendered sketches.

Drawing is both the act of rendering what you see into an image, **and an ability to portray things that your mind can see, but which do not yet exist.** There is joy to be had in the improvement of consistent practice, and drawing may help you think more clearly.

One of the more illuminating exercises is to draw your own self-portrait while you go through a drawing course, and to see it improve.

Commitment: Read *Drawing On The Right Side Of The Brain.* Work through the exercises, and see how your perception of the world changes.

Journal...

Don't Bite Your Fingernails

"I bite the hell out of my fingernails. I can't stop. I should stop. It would be nice to grow my fingernails out. It would be healthier. I could pick up dimes." – Jackie Earle Haley

To-Do's
✔
✔
✔
✔
✔
✔

The nail-biters among us do it for many reasons, but there are no good ones. There are better ways to alleviate stress. Better nervous habits that are easier on our teeth, cuticles, and that aren't considered impolite behavior. Easier said than done if you're a chronic nail-biter, but there is no downside to breaking this habit.

One of the easiest ways to stop is to clip your fingernails regularly. Then you're never in danger of looking down, being embarrassed at the state of your nails, and gnawing them off before anyone notices how long they are. You can also wear nail polish, whose nasty taste should dissuade you.

Commitment: Stop biting your nails. Treat yourself to an expensive manicure that you would never consider munching on.

Long-Term Goals

☐ ☐ ☐ ☐ ☐ ☐

Journal...

Write A Poem

"Poetry is an echo, asking a shadow to dance." – Carl Sandburg

To-Do's		Long-Term Goals

There is a style of poetry that nearly everyone can find a way to enjoy. If you groan at the thought of an epic like *The Faerie Queene* or *Paradise Lost,* you might enjoy the beats. If you can't stand the beats, you might like the modernists. If you can't stand any of it, you might like Shel Silverstein and Dr. Seuss.

There's no wrong way to read, or enjoy poetry. *Or* to write it. And writing a poem can be a fun and enriching challenge, whether you read anyone else's poems or not. **Poetry forces you to slow down and really focus on what you want to convey**, whether it's an image, a feeling, or a simple rhyme scheme for fun.

You can't just start typing at full-bore and expect a poem to appear. But poetry can be as simple as precise reductionism.

Commitment: Write a poem this week. Don't take it too seriously.

Journal...

Learn An Instrument

"One good thing about music, when it hits you, you feel no pain." – Bob Marley

To-Do's		Long-Term Goals

I once heard of a ninety-nine-year-old woman who decided to start taking piano lessons. Why? Because she had always wanted to. We're not all going to be prodigies, but it's never too late to learn an instrument.

Simply put, there's really nothing like being able to use your hands and breath to make music. Sit down with a guitar, and whether you're playing a basic A Major scale or you're ripping away at a flamenco piece that would make everyone want to dance, **you're making music that *would not exist without you.***

Music is calming, and the practice of an instrument can work wonders for confidence. It's very difficult to practice and not improve, and with an instrument, the improvement means you can play better music, or write it.

Commitment: What's your favorite instrument? See if you can get one, grab yourself an easy practice book, and see if you like it. Youtube videos on lessons. Eventually hire a teacher.

Journal...

Use Your Public Library

"If you have a garden and a library, you have everything you need." – Marcus Tullius Cicero

To-Do's
✔
✔
✔
✔
✔
✔

The library means different things to different people. Perhaps it is a place where you get your books. Maybe you haven't been back since childhood. Maybe you avoided the library entirely because you didn't like to read, or thought you didn't. Maybe you take your kids there for storytimes.

Libraries have changed. They're not just the buildings with the books anymore. They offer programs, speakers, trivia nights, databases for researching everything from Photoshop to stock investing, and much more.

A library card is free. Its value cannot be measured once you find your own reason to use your library.

Commitment: Visit your library. See what's new. Get a library card. Commit to saving money by using the library instead of Amazon.

Long-Term Goals
☐
☐
☐
☐
☐
☐

Journal...

_____

Picture Food In Its Original State

"Clean, tasty, real foods do not come processed in boxes or bags; they come from the earth, the sea, the field, or the farm." – Suzanne Somers

To-Do's		Long-Term Goals

✔

✔

✔

✔

✔

✔

✔

It's never a bad idea to question the composition of the food we eat. No one sets out to eat a bunch of harmful toxins, or even trace amounts of the bad stuff, but it can still happen.

One easy guideline you can use to make sure you're eating healthier is to try this simple visualization. Look at what you're about to eat. Can you picture it in its original state? If you're looking at a banana, then yes. It grew on a tree somewhere. We all know where acorns and cashews come from. The same is true with a steak or a fillet of fish.

But, a twinkie? A bag of chips? Do you really know how it all started and what had to happen for it to arrive at your mouth in its current shape, bag, and flavor? Probably not.

Commitment: If you can't picture what your food looked like in its original state, pass on it. It's not food. It won't nourish your body.

☐
☐
☐
☐
☐
☐
☐

Journal...

Don't Waste Food

"Wasting food is like stealing from the poor." – Pope Francis

To-Do's		Long-Term Goals

To-Do's
- ✔
- ✔
- ✔
- ✔
- ✔
- ✔
- ✔
- ✔

"There are people starving who would be grateful for that," is a common refrain at dinner tables in America, usually when a child who is a picky eater is turning up his or her nose at something. And, while this is true, the lesson doesn't always seem to sink in.

Do you clean your plate every time? Give yourself smaller portions. Do you ever have to toss something from the back of the fridge out because you forgot about it and it went bad before you could finish it? Cook less next time. Do you discard something as soon as it's a tiny bit stale? Buy smaller quantities.

Keep the perspective that **there are in fact people, who go to bed hungry,** but who could have eaten what many of us throw away, whether we do so out of obliviousness or carelessness. The least we can do is to simply eat what we buy or cook.

Commitment: No more wasted food. Think about better uses for leftovers. Or better yet, avoid having leftovers in the first place.

Long-Term Goals
- ☐
- ☐
- ☐
- ☐
- ☐
- ☐
- ☐
- ☐

Journal...

Wash Your Dishes

"I have to admit that I'm one of those people that thinks the dishwasher is a miracle." – Clarence Thomas

To-Do's		Long-Term Goals

Germs are everywhere. *Everywhere.* And the best chance you have of fighting them is not letting them propagate unnecessarily. One of the easiest ways to do this is to wash your dishes *thoroughly.* I wouldn't be surprised if there are college dorms where forks get the "Just a rinse" treatments for months on end.

No no no! Even if you don't have a dishwasher, dishes need to be washed in hot water, with soap. It's not the most convenient chore, and it's no adrenaline rush, but the costs of putting dirty dishware into your mouth, or setting your food on it, over and over, far outweigh the couple of extra minutes it will take to wash thoroughly.

Commitment: If you're not washing your dishes as well as you could, start immediately. Invest in nice sponges and good soap. Use dishwashing as playtime with your youngest kids. They love to help out.

Journal...

July

July 1

Get Handier

"Not only do I know how to milk a cow, but I know how to herd a bunch of cows, too, which is a life skill that I think may come in handy someday." – Martina McBride

To-Do's		Long-Term Goals

You may never need to milk a cow, or herd a bunch of them, but there are basic skills that every adult should know. It's true, some of us have mechanical aptitudes that others do not, but we can all be handier than we are.

Do you know where the fusebox is in your house? Do you know how to locate the struts? Do you know how to shut off a leaky pipe? Can you use a power drill? Would you know how to hang a picture, or which fasteners can be used to anchor a picture into different sorts of walls? These are just a few of the many, many examples we could talk about.

Start small. Think about the things that you currently need other people to do for you. Which of them do you think you could learn to do?

Commitment: Begin learning one new handy skill this week. Keep going until you have confidence in your ability, then add another to your toolbox.

Journal...

Maintain Your Automobile

"I'd ban all automobiles from the central part of the city. You see, the automobile was just a passing fad. It's got to go. It's got to go a long way from here." – Lawrence Ferlinghetti

To-Do's
✔
✔
✔
✔
✔
✔
✔

Unless you don't drive, and you also live somewhere where the automobile does not exist, then these incredible devices are part of your life. If you rely on a car or truck for your transportation, then you probably know the misery that results from getting stuck when a car breaks down, or the pain of shelling out your money for a costly repair.

As with all machines, automobiles will just break down sometimes. But there are things we can do to make sure this doesn't happen more often than it needs to.

Learn (and practice) basic car maintenance. Get your oil changed when you should. Keep the proper amount of air in your tires. Keep your fluids topped off. Learn how to change a tire. This will spare you a lot of headaches. **It's the small things in life, which we neglect, that can cause a lot of unexpected misery.**

Commitment: Learn and practice basic car maintenance. Take an automotive class at the local community college.

Long-Term Goals

☐
☐
☐
☐
☐
☐
☐

Journal...

July 3

Do Not Cheat On Your Significant Other

"There's so many different ways to cheat. People think infidelity is the way to cheat. I think it's sometimes far worse to emotionally cheat on somebody." – Sandra Bullock

To-Do's		Long-Term Goals

Let's be very clear. Cheating on your significant other is never justifiable, regardless of who is in the right or wrong. Even if your partner forgives you in the aftermath, even if your partner was not fulfilling their end of the relationship contract, there is no way to say that cheating is a just act.

Trust takes a lifetime to create, but only a second to destroy. And this is the true victim of infidelity. Not all problems have a solution. But cheating is *never* a real solution. It is a shortcut, and often serves as a tailor-made crisis, which can then precipitate the end of the relationship.

If you need someone else besides your partner, then there is probably someone else for you. But have the integrity to end it with your partner before you move to someone else.

Commitment: If you're thinking about cheating, pause for a second and ask yourself why. At the end of the day, the act will define you much more than it does your partner.

Journal...

Be An Informed Citizen

"National security laws must protect national security. But they must also protect the public trust and preserve the ability of an informed electorate to hold its government to account." – Al Franken

To-Do's		Long-Term Goals

Wherever you live, it is a good idea—although it might be better viewed as a duty—to pay attention to what is happening in your country. To what is happening with your government. **Political outrage is cheap and easy** and can even be fun in its own perverse way, but multitudes of people in America are shockingly ill-informed on the issues they say matter most to them.

Being an informed citizen is necessary for becoming an ideal citizen, meaning, a citizen with educated opinions, the conviction to speak up when something is wrong or could be improved civically, and a willingness to participate in the governance of a country.

If we do not understand the issues and challenges facing a town, state, or country, we forfeit the right to some of our reaction when the people who do understand make choices without us.

Commitment: Read at least one local and one national newspaper every day.

Journal...

Eat More Raw Food

"Life is too short not to eat raw and it's even shorter if you don't." – Marie Sarantakis

To-Do's

- ✔
- ✔
- ✔
- ✔
- ✔
- ✔
- ✔

Long-Term Goals

- ☐
- ☐
- ☐
- ☐
- ☐
- ☐
- ☐

The ethics of vegetarianism and veganism are beyond the scope of this book. But regardless of how you approach food from an ethical standpoint, **there are indisputable health benefits to a plant-based diet.**

"Eat your vegetables" is a bit of health advice you probably started hearing back in grade school. It is almost impossible to eat too many vegetables, and the statistics on how many people do not eat enough vegetables are sobering. Unless you are a vegetarian, the chances that you're getting as many vegetables as you should be are slim, unless you're in the veggie-happy minority.

So start small. Eat *more* vegetables. Just more. Then start scaling up.

Commitment: Just make sure you're getting vegetables with every meal. Read *Proteinholic* by Dr. Gath Davis, a fellow bariatric surgeon.

Journal...

Ask People Good Questions

"Good Questions Outrank Easy Answers." – Paul Samuelson

To-Do's

- ✔
- ✔
- ✔
- ✔
- ✔
- ✔
- ✔
- ✔
- ✔

Long-Term Goals

- ☐
- ☐
- ☐
- ☐
- ☐
- ☐
- ☐
- ☐
- ☐

One of the easiest and most natural ways to build rapport with people is to ask them questions. *Good* questions. Meaning, questions that will allow them to open up about themselves and talk about their passions and goals. **The best questions are often open-ended, and offer opportunities for tangents and introspection.**

For instance, if someone asks you, "What were your challenges this week?" it's a big question that might take some thought as you figure out how to answer it. You might not even have thought about your challenges until prompted to think about it.

Think about first-date chit chat. "What's your job? Do you like it?" Stuff like that. Once you're past the getting to know you stage, truly getting a glimpse of who someone is, goes beyond the harmless, easy, low stakes conversations of first dates. Ask questions in a way that will really let people think and talk. This will also make you a better listener.

Commitment: The next time you're with someone, ask them deeper questions than you usually would, and really listen to what they say.

Journal...

Learn To Listen

"One of the most sincere forms of respect is actually listening to what another has to say." – Bryant H. McGill

To-Do's		**Long-Term Goals**

Do you think that you are a good listener? Perhaps this is a better question—would the people around you say that you're a good listener? There's a big difference between hearing and listening. If you've ever felt like you are not being listened to, you know this difference well.

Listening means paying attention, not just waiting for your turn to speak. Listening means trying to empathize with and understand what the person is saying, so you can respond in the most useful way, not in a way that you've already planned to.

Most importantly, **listening requires effort and a willingness to slow down,** and that's the sticking point for many of us.

Commitment: Make the effort to listen. This week, start small and simply commit to listening more than you speak. The Dalai Lama said, "When you talk, you are repeating what you already know. But when you listen, you may learn something new."

Journal...

Practice Generosity

"Generosity is giving more than you can, and pride is taking less than you need." – Khalil Gibran

To-Do's
✔
✔
✔
✔
✔
✔
✔

You never know just how far a little kindness or encouragement will go in another person's day. **And you'll never hear from many of the people you can help through small acts of generosity.** But if you've ever been cheered up by someone's unexpected generosity, you know the difference you could make for someone else.

Time is the most precious resource we have, and time is often what is most appreciated. Listening takes time. Getting to know someone takes time. Being a shoulder to cry on takes time. Helping someone feel less lonely takes time. And each moment we spend on someone else is a moment of generosity.

Commitment: Find one opportunity each day to practice generosity. Start with your family, your inner circle. Note the acts of generosity in your journal, even though you might never hear about them.

Long-Term Goals

☐
☐
☐
☐
☐
☐
☐

Journal...

Make Eye Contact

"I have a big thing with eye contact, because I think as soon as you make eye contact with somebody, you see them, and they become valued and worthy." – Mary Lambert

To-Do's

✔

✔

✔

✔

✔

✔

✔

✔

✔

How do you feel when someone won't meet your eyes? Like, ever? Most of us have probably known someone like this. Maybe some of us have been (or are still) that person. It feels like the person is shy, or afraid, or like they're just being crushed by life, or that they have no confidence, or that they're maladjusted. All of the above, or none of the above, but it's a sign of *something*.

Eye contact shows confidence. This is why most dating guides instruct people to make eye contact with potential partners who they are interested in getting to know. Eye contact shows interest, and not everyone is comfortable with it. You've probably heard the old chestnut that "eyes are the windows to the soul." Well, assume that it's true for a moment. **How well will you get to know someone if you can't even look into their eyes?** Conversely, how will they ever get to know you?

One caveat: don't stare. Staring is hostile and creepy. Make consistent, confident eye contact with people when you speak with them, but take breaks. Blink. Act natural.

Commitment: This week, make eye contact more than you're used to. People will respond to you differently, and you will have a chance at strengthening the bonds you already have.

Long-Term Goals

☐

☐

☐

☐

☐

☐

☐

☐

☐

☐

Journal...

Read The Bible (At Least Once)

"God writes the Gospel not in the Bible alone, but also on trees, and in the flowers and clouds and stars." –
Martin Luther

To-Do's
✔
✔
✔
✔
✔
✔
✔

Whether you believe in it or not, it's hard to make a case for a book being more influential than The Bible. Reading a book that is considered sacred by hundreds of millions of people, across millennia, is always an education, whether it be a spiritual education, an exercise in comparative religion, or a head-scratching slog.

The Bible has immeasurable influence on the world we live in and the people in our communities. **To understand it is to have a better understanding of the world we live in.**

The same goes for The Koran, The Talmud, and any other books of scripture that continue to have import for modern life.

Commitment: Read the Bible at least once in your life without judgment. If it's interesting to you, write down any observations you have.

Long-Term Goals
☐
☐
☐
☐
☐
☐
☐

Journal...

_____
_____
_____
_____
_____
_____
_____
_____
_____
_____
_____
_____
_____
_____
_____
_____
_____
_____
_____
_____
_____
_____
_____

Avoid Assumptions

"Assumptions are the termites of relationships." – Henry Winkler

To-Do's		Long-Term Goals

A man was out of breath at an intersection, waiting for the light to turn green so he could continue his run. Utterly spent, he was bent at the waist with his head nearly between his knees. A car pulled up and the window rolled down. "Looks like you should give up running!" yelled a voice from within.

What the person in the car didn't know was that the runner was in training for a marathon. He had just finished the nineteenth mile of a grueling practice run. He had logged over a hundred miles of running in the previous ten days.

It sounds trite, but things are not always what they seem. **To make an assumption on incomplete information is to hazard a guess.** And when you guess, you can guess wrong. Really wrong.

Commitment: Avoid making assumptions. Strive to be more open-minded.

Journal...

Read An Audiobook

"There are three kinds of men. The one that learns by reading. The few who learn by observation. The rest of them have to pee on the electric fence for themselves." — Will Rogers

To-Do's		Long-Term Goals

First of all, let go of the idea that listening to a book is a lesser form of reading. Books are made of words and ideas, and words and ideas retain their meaning whether they are heard or seen.

But this is where *certain* audiobooks can be the wrong choice for a particular reader. It's hard not to zone out occasionally during an audiobook, whether it's for ten seconds or two minutes. If you're listening to a propulsive thriller and your only job is to follow the storyline, you probably can jump right back in. If you're listening to something dense, academic, philosophical, and/or full of terms you're unfamiliar with, maybe you can't afford to miss a minute of the listen.

Listening to books is a way to sneak in a dozen or more books a year than you'd get to otherwise, even if you just listen to them during a commute to work or to the grocery store.

Commitment: Listen to an audiobook. Choose one that you can absorb, and whose subject you won't lose when you run into the inevitable moments of distraction that pop up while listening. I listen to self-help audiobooks at 1.5x or 2x the normal speed. This tip really accelerated my learning.

Journal...

Letting Go Of Should

"If you take responsibility for yourself you will develop a hunger to accomplish your dreams." – Les Brown

To-Do's

✔

✔

✔

✔

✔

✔

Long-Term Goals

☐
☐
☐
☐
☐
☐

It can be hard at times to know what we need to do with our own lives, to say nothing of the extra responsibility of pretending to know what other people should do with theirs. And yet, it's easy to catch ourselves telling someone else what he or she "should" do, or talking about what "should" happen.

"Should" pretends at a moral certainty that we may not be qualified to give when it comes to another person. "Could" makes a lot more sense, is a lot more honest, and leaves the possibility of doubt. It reminds us that unpredictability is a fact of life, and that, no matter how we think things should be, we don't always get our way.

Commitment: Pay attention to how often you talk about how things should be, or what people should do. Replace it with could and see if it changes your perspective.

Journal...

Improve Your Grammar

"Grammar is a piano I play by ear. All I know about grammar is its power." – Joan Didion

To-Do's

- ✓
- ✓
- ✓
- ✓
- ✓
- ✓
- ✓
- ✓
- ✓

Long-Term Goals

- ☐
- ☐
- ☐
- ☐
- ☐
- ☐
- ☐
- ☐
- ☐

Grammar is not just a tool that nit-picky professors and teachers use to torment their students. All communication relies on the clarity of a message being expressed between two parties. Think about verbal communication. There are factors outside of the words being said that can change the reception of the message. Demeanor, delivery, tone of voice, etc.

In writing, poor grammar can give the person you're trying to communicate with a reason to dismiss, ignore, or question what you are trying to say, simply because of how you are saying it. There are exceptions, of course. If you're texting with a friend and you're both used to typing "ur" for "you are," then no one else gets to say anything about it.

But if you're writing any sort of professional correspondence, or applying for a job, or pitching a magazine article, or writing a grant, you will give readers who read with an eye to dismiss—often to reduce their workload and save time—a reason to dismiss you.

Commitment: Improving grammar doesn't need to be a misery. Pick up a copy of *Eats, Shoots, And Leaves* by Lynne Truss. Use an online grammar aid before you submit your writing.

Journal...

_____
_____
_____
_____
_____
_____
_____
_____
_____
_____
_____
_____
_____
_____
_____
_____
_____
_____
_____
_____
_____

Not Everyone Will Like You—And That's Okay

"There're two people in the world that are not likeable: a master and a slave." – Nikki Giovanni

To-Do's		Long-Term Goals

✔

✔

✔

✔

✔

✔

✔

✔

✔

It is nice to be liked and it can really be a bummer when someone doesn't like you. And yet, it might not be about you at all when you just feel like you rub someone the wrong way. Simply trying to get along with everyone is not a goal worth aspiring to, because following your own convictions and beliefs will inevitably put you at odds with people who do not share them.

Think about this: **What do you get out of being liked?** Why do you want people to like you? For many people, the fact that someone doesn't like them produces a worry—or worse, they take it as proof—that they are not likable. Being liked is validating, but it's not as useful or important as liking yourself first.

If you are happy with yourself and the direction you are pursuing, the opinions of others will have less sway over you. And the chances are, if you meet someone who truly doesn't like you, you're probably not going to have to spend a lot of time together anyway.

Commitment: Like yourself first, and you will handle it better when someone else fails to take a shine to you.

□

□

□

□

□

□

□

□

□

Journal...

Check Your Email Less

"Email is familiar. It's comfortable. It's easy to use. But it might just be the biggest killer of time and productivity in the office today." – Ryan Holmes

To-Do's
✔
✔
✔
✔
✔
✔
✔
✔
✔
✔

Email can be a great tool. It can also be a massive time waster, even when used with the best intentions. Now that just about everyone has a smartphone, it's become possible to check email incessantly. **Actually, it might be more accurate to say that for many people it's become impossible *not* to check email incessantly.**

How many of us actually work in such a high-pressure, high-stakes field that we *must* be responding to emails, or writing them, or checking to see if we have any new message, every five minutes? If you're one of the compulsive email checkers, would things be *so* dire if you checked email five times a day? Or three? Or...one?

It will vary from case to case. But it is almost certainly true that most of us can check email less than we do. Checking and responding to a block of emails all at once uses less time than constantly returning to an email account just to see what's going on. And it mitigates the diffusion of focus that occurs when we're trying to multitask too much. When it's time to do email, do it. When it's not, don't even try.

Commitment: Check your email half as often over the next week as you're used to. Set a limit for yourself. Be consistent with the times you check email. If you do this and there's no catastrophic fallout, consider cutting back even more.

Long-Term Goals
☐
☐
☐
☐
☐
☐
☐
☐
☐
☐

Journal...

_____
_____
_____
_____
_____
_____
_____
_____
_____
_____
_____
_____
_____
_____
_____
_____
_____
_____

Switch Sides

"You can't just carry everyone else's hopes and fears around in your backpack and expect to stand up straight."
– David Kirk

To-Do's		Long-Term Goals

Whether you carry a purse, a briefcase, a backpack, or a messenger back, chances are you favor one side. These aren't the heaviest items in the world, but over time, if you put all of the extra weight on one shoulder or arm or hand, it *will* change your posture.

It just takes awareness to switch off. If you wore a purse over your right shoulder today, choose the left tomorrow. Ditto with all of the other accessories or bags you can carry or wear. These asymmetrical changes creep up in degrees, so you may not notice that your posture has altered until someone points it out. **And every imbalance you pick up makes it easier to pick up other imbalances.**

Switching sides is a really easy change to make that will keep you evened out and spare you other potential pain.

Commitment: Just change shoulders or hands regularly. Every other time is ideal.

Journal...

Give Speed Reading a Try

"I am not a speed reader. I am a speed understander." – Isaac Asimov

To-Do's

- ✔
- ✔
- ✔
- ✔
- ✔
- ✔
- ✔
- ✔
- ✔
- ✔
- ✔
- ✔

Long-Term Goals

- ☐
- ☐
- ☐
- ☐
- ☐
- ☐
- ☐
- ☐
- ☐
- ☐
- ☐
- ☐

Did you ever see a speed-reading infomercial? They usually involved someone "reading" a book as fast as you could flip a page, often while dragging a finger across the lines before setting the book down, 90 seconds later, and proclaiming "done!" before the product barkers would give the price point. It would be nice to read a dozen books a day, but the claims weren't always on the level.

However, speed-reading is real. **Reading is a skill, and anything that can be practiced can be improved.** Sometimes being improved means an increase in speed, but not always. Speed-reading is the art of 1) training the eyes to take in more words at a glance while allowing the eyes to stop fewer times per sentence; 2) the art of eliminating the "internal voice" that reads along with you in your head.

Both can be done; they just require practice. It is worth asking, though, what might be lost in the process. It is possible to increase the amount of words you can see and comprehend at ever-greater speeds. This technique is great for self-help books. But is this how you want to read a beautiful piece of writing? There's no time in speed-reading to enjoy an elegant turn of phrase or shiver in recognition over a perfect metaphor. And good luck speed-reading a dense philosophical text whose every sentence might require unpacking before proceeding. But see for yourself.

Commitment: Get a copy of Evelyn Wood's Speed Reading Program and give yourself a few practice sessions. Your ability will improve. Then you can decide if it's a style of reading you enjoy.

Journal...

_____
_____
_____
_____
_____
_____
_____
_____
_____
_____
_____
_____
_____
_____
_____

Map It Out

"If geography is prose, maps are iconography." – Lennart Meri

To-Do's

✔

✔

✔

✔

✔

✔

✔

✔

Long-Term Goals

☐

☐

☐

☐

☐

☐

☐

☐

For many of us, geography meant learning state capitals, and maybe how to point to all of the states on a US map, if our teachers were particularly ambitious. But there's a big world out there, and sadly, there don't seem to be many people who know where much of anything is.

You may never run into a situation where someone says, "Hey! Point to Laos on a map or else!" But it's hard to say that there's a downside to knowing where things are, particularly if you're interested in current events. Much foreign policy comes about simply because of where countries and people lie in relation to one another.

Understanding the world means understanding what is in the world. And understanding where things are will enrich that understanding. It will ignite your desire to travel more and see some of the world's great natural wonders that you've only been reading about.

Commitment: There are a lot of wonderful, free geography apps and online games that can teach you the world's countries in a couple of weeks or less. Get one. Use it.

Journal...

Walk On The Balls Of Your Feet

"You don't live in a castle full of spiral stairs without getting calves of adamantium." – Lev Grossman

To-Do's		Long-Term Goals

✔

✔

✔

✔

✔

✔

✔

✔

This tip concerns those of you who would like shapelier and better-defined calve muscles. Have you ever taken a look at a troupe of ballerinas? As willowy and svelte as they are, their calves are probably impressive. It's because they're always up on their toes.

Don't panic. Nobody is suggesting that you buy ballet flats and get up on your toes. But maybe try walking on the balls of your feet whenever you're able, and see if your leg muscles don't fall in line with some diligence. It can take a surprising amount of concentration and strength, and depending on how weak or strong the ankles are, many people learn that they can't even raise up all the way onto the balls of their feet.

Commitment: Whenever you can remember—and maybe when nobody's looking, if you're self-conscious—walk on the balls of your feet. Try to increase the time, or the amount of time, that you spend on your toes each day. Start by doing it whenever you're walking from your living room to the kitchen or bathroom.

☐
☐
☐
☐
☐
☐
☐
☐

Journal...

Watch Your Heels

"To be happy, it first takes being comfortable being in your own shoes. The rest can work up from there." –
Sophia Bush

To-Do's		Long-Term Goals

It doesn't take long to start seeing wear on a pair of new shoes, particularly if you have any ankle or feet issues that cause you to walk on the edges of your feet. For people whose feet evert badly—think feet that are pointing slightly past the "10 and 2" position on a clock—often wind up walking on the edges of their feet so drastically that the outer half of the heel wears away.

Take a look at the heels of an old shoe and you will learn much about how the wearer walks. Learn some basic biomechanics and the heels of someone's shoes will give you a glimpse of just how much discomfort the wearer is in, or will be.

Commitment: Pay attention to your heels. If you can't change your gait, rotate your shoes through often enough so that you're always walking on a relatively level heel. Go to a professional running store, so they can test your gait and recommend shoe inserts as needed.

Journal...

Ditch The Kids' Cereal

"Like religion, politics, and family planning, cereal is not a topic to be brought up in public. It's too controversial." – Erma Bombeck

To-Do's
✔
✔
✔
✔
✔
✔

It can be hard not to get nostalgic for childhood mornings with a bowl of cereal that was basically candy. Sitting down with a bowl of Apple Jacks or Captain Crunch to start the day felt like a reward just for waking up. **Of course, it wasn't healthy for us as children, but we could get away with it.**

And obviously, it's not healthy for us as adults. Breakfast sets you up for the day, and it's worth doing right. But, just like you wouldn't get up and eat a bowlful of sugar in order to prepare yourself for a productive day of life, you might want to reconsider the sugary kids' cereals in the same light, if you're still eating them.

Commitment: Switch to a healthy cereal to stop your habit. Eventually graduate to healthy green smoothies.

Long-Term Goals

☐ ☐ ☐ ☐ ☐ ☐

Journal...

July 23

Tell People You Love Them

"Cherish your human connections - your relationships with friends and family." – Barbara Bush

To-Do's

- ✔
- ✔
- ✔
- ✔
- ✔
- ✔
- ✔
- ✔

Long-Term Goals

- ☐
- ☐
- ☐
- ☐
- ☐
- ☐
- ☐
- ☐
- ☐

Life is short. Sad but true. And not everyone will be lucky enough to have people they love, and who love them, during their lifetimes. For those of us who are lucky enough, we should remind these people that we love them every chance we get. **None of us knows when we'll see someone for the last time.**

When we think of the final words we might say to someone, is there anything better, or more memorable, than "I love you?" No matter how long we live, we will only have so many chances to say it.

You don't need to stumble around, maudlin in the face of our mortality, proclaiming your love for all man night and day, but when you can do it sincerely, tell the people who you actually love. Don't assume they know, or that they won't enjoy hearing it. Tell them. Also, this means you'll hear it said back to you more often.

Commitment: The next time you see a friend or family member, tell them that you love them. Make a promise that "I love you" will be the last thing you say to end every conversation with your loved one because one day, it will be.

Journal...

Learn About Your Heritage

"Your ancestors are rooting for you." – Eleanor Brownn

To-Do's

- ✔
- ✔
- ✔
- ✔
- ✔
- ✔
- ✔
- ✔

Long-Term Goals

- ☐
- ☐
- ☐
- ☐
- ☐
- ☐
- ☐
- ☐

Every one of us is part of a story that began when our parents met, and when theirs met, and all the way on back. **Learning your family history can be an amazing ride.** How much do you truly know about your parents? About your grandparents? Once you start looking, assuming you have access to their information, you will gain a new appreciation for them.

But it isn't just a matter of sentiment. Wherever you live, if you're the parents of immigrants, you are part of another country's heritage as well. It might not be part of your hardwiring, but the chances of you finding something interesting while researching that country are pretty high.

Make notes of the family stories you find that you like the most. You are here because of all the family members who came before you and their experiences.

Commitment: Go to a family history library, or a genealogy website, and start working backwards. Enjoy the trip and try to feel the connection with the family chain that produced you.

Journal...

Use Conditioner

"I have so much residue crap in my hair from years and years of not washing it and not having any sense of personal hygiene whatsoever. Even today, I go into these things where I'm supposed to be this sexy guy or whatever, and I'm literally asking, 'If I get plumes of dandruff on me, can you just brush it off?'" – Robert Pattinson

To-Do's

- ✔
- ✔
- ✔
- ✔
- ✔
- ✔

You don't have to have a full head of commercial-quality hair in order to use conditioner. You just have to want to avoid a dry scalp full of flakes. There are plenty of bald guys out there who can still benefit from conditioner, even though "washing their hair" basically means "washing their heads."

Conditioner doesn't take long to use. You just rub some in your hair and let it sit for a couple of minutes in the shower. You can also try leave-in conditioners. Then you don't have to deal with a dry scalp that is constantly leaving a trail in your wake and settling onto your shoulders.

Commitment: Use conditioner, whether you're down to stubble or you've got a head of hair that Pantene would pay for.

Long-Term Goals

- ☐
- ☐
- ☐
- ☐
- ☐
- ☐

Journal...

Don't Be A Victim

"Never be bullied into silence. Never allow yourself to be made a victim. Accept no one's definition of your life; define yourself." – Harvey Fierstein

To-Do's		Long-Term Goals

When Victor Frankl was a prisoner in a Nazi death camp, he decided that the only thing he could control were his reactions to his situation. If he wanted to live—and he did— he had to admit that he had no control over his body or his time, or what the Nazis chose to do with his body, and the schedule they exerted over his time. **But he could control his mind.**

In unimaginable circumstances, he chose to stay positive. He was the very *definition* of a victim—the monstrosity of the Holocaust perpetrated on the Jewish people was the very definition of victimization—but Frankl would not be broken by it. If he chose to see himself as a victim, he'd start thinking like a victim, and if he started thinking like a victim, he would start acting like a victim.

If he found a way to escape the trap of victimhood, we all can.

Commitment: Read *Man's Search For Meaning* by Victor Frankl. It's a short book that you will never forget.

Journal...

Thoughts Become Actions

"A strong, successful man is not the victim of his environment. He creates favorable conditions. His own inherent force and energy compel things to turn out as he desires." – Orison Swett Marden

To-Do's		Long-Term Goals

You don't have to look very far to find an article, video, book, or person who will tell you that visualizing success is essential for success. On the flipside, you probably won't find the article, video, book, or person who is going to tell you that visualizing failure is essential for failure. But we do it anyway, even if we aren't aware of it in such stark terms.

Thoughts lead to actions. If your thoughts are about failure—whether your own or someone else's failure—ask yourself what the point is? What actions will those thoughts lead to? If you are naturally a negative person, you probably don't give yourself many chances to think positively. **If your thoughts produce your actions, at the very least, negative thoughts are going to lead you to inaction.**

Commitment: Become more aware of your thoughts. Observe yourself for a day and try to decide, roughly, the ratio of your negative to positive thoughts. Then start working in the right direction.

Journal...

Don't Live Small To Make Other People Comfortable

"Truth is a point of view, but authenticity can't be faked." – Peter Gruber

To-Do's		Long-Term Goals

✔

✔

✔

✔

✔

✔

✔

Let's be clear: Arrogance is real. Showing off is an unworthy behavior. But a lot of people who lack confidence see *all* confidence as arrogance. They can see any demonstration of talent or ability as showing off. There's nothing wrong with wanting to be humble, but you are under no obligation to hide your talents or skills or appearance or good fortune solely so that insecure people can feel more secure.

Do not live a smaller life so that people can feel better about themselves. Your time on this rotating blue sphere has a limited number of revolutions. Don't antagonize and brag and bluster, but you have every right to be proud of yourself and to act like it.

And consider this—your confidence may inspire someone else to act more confident.

Commitment: Know the difference between arrogant and confident. When you're sure that you're not arrogant, be confident and never apologize for it.

☐ ☐ ☐ ☐ ☐ ☐ ☐

Journal...

Stop Waiting

"Every bad situation is a blues song waiting to happen." – Amy Winehouse

To-Do's		Long-Term Goals

Part of living in the moment means not simply waiting for things to change. There's a bit of a high-wire act going on here, because our positive actions now do have the potential to make our futures better, but the focus—unless you're doing something reckless where it would be better to delay your gratification—should be on the moment.

Don't wait for things to get better, or to be different. If you know an avenue you can try, try it. Remember, what we dream up as a worst case scenario is usually unlikely, and not all that bad to begin with, if we have the proper perspective.

John Lennon said life is what happens while you're making other plans. If not now, when? Why are you hesitant? Behind hesitancy, there is fear. **Like kerosene to a bonfire, the fuel for fear is time.** Therefore, the longer you wait, the more afraid you will become.

Commitment: Stop waiting. If you know what you want, move on it. Remember, fear loves time.

Journal...

There's Nothing Special About Being Busy

"The way to get started is to quit talking and begin doing." – Walt Disney

To-Do's		Long-Term Goals

There's a difference between productivity and business. It isn't hard to be busy, and it's even easier to look busy. You just furrow your brow, move fast, look at your watch with an impatient expression on your face, and voila! But the idea that busyness for its own sake is useful, or a sign of a hard worker, is nonsense.

For each of us, our busyness should contribute to the things that are most important to us. Sure, if you do a ton of work in a day, you were productive; but if you didn't produce things that are important to *you,* you might as well have just been busy.

This is a matter of perspective. You're not automatically working hard because you're busy, and you're not necessarily taking it easy if you're not busy. **Results are what matter most, and results are the realm of productivity.**

Commitment: Be productive, not just busy. You know the difference. Produce results that matter to you.

Journal...

Detach From Outcomes

"Nothing is perfect. Life is messy. Relationships are complex. Outcomes are uncertain. People are irrational." –
Hugh Mackay

To-Do's		Long-Term Goals
✔	This is a tip about what our goals mean to us. We set them, we pursue them, and still, there are going to be times when we fall short. Maybe we were unrealistic. Maybe circumstances changed, or our ideals did. There are a lot of things that can derail the pursuit of a goal.	☐
✔		☐
✔	If that happens, no matter how diligently you were pursuing the goal, it's best if the disappointment doesn't break you. It sounds contradictory, but we should both pursue our goals single-mindedly *and* not attribute too much importance to their outcomes. **It is not the achievement of the goal that is important, but rather what we become in the process that matters most.**	☐
✔		☐
✔		☐
✔	It is possible to think a goal means more than it does.	☐

Commitment: Detach your sense of self-worth from outcomes and focus instead on the journey.

Journal...

August

Let People Make Their Own First Impressions

"Don't live up to your stereotypes." – Sherman Alexie

To-Do's

- ✔
- ✔
- ✔
- ✔
- ✔
- ✔
- ✔
- ✔

Long-Term Goals

- ☐
- ☐
- ☐
- ☐
- ☐
- ☐
- ☐
- ☐

It's an old joke that stereotypes are great time savers. The joke lies in the fact that stereotyping someone requires you to assume that you already know the most important thing about the person, simply because of their gender, ethnicity, beliefs, occupation, etc.

Think about what you like about yourself, and what you wish people knew about you. Now imagine that every time someone saw you for the first time, or read your demographic info, they thought they already knew everything about you that mattered. There wouldn't be anything you could say, and no way to persuade them that there's more to you.

It's an awful thought, and no one should ever have to be in that position. We each deserve to make our own first impressions, and we must allow others to do the same.

Commitment: Have a very honest conversation with yourself about whether you stereotype anyone. Try not to assign qualities to someone based on race, religion, gender, etc...give them the dignity to make their own first impression.

Journal...

_____
_____
_____
_____
_____
_____
_____
_____
_____
_____
_____
_____
_____
_____
_____
_____
_____
_____
_____
_____
_____
_____
_____

Park As Far Away From The Door As You Can

"Take care of your body. It's the only place you have to live." – Jim Rohn

To-Do's		Long-Term Goals

✔

✔

✔

✔

✔

✔

✔

This one doesn't take a lot of explanation. If you drive, that means you eventually park your car. When you park your car, you should park as far away from the door as possible. Just in case the reason isn't clear, it's so that you will do a little more walking than you would if you parked closer to the door.

At the gym, at the grocery store, at home, any time you can add a few steps to your walk, you'll make a tiny investment in your overall health and mobility. There are exceptions, of course. Don't park a mile away from the grocery store if you're in a hurry. Don't park so far away from work that you're late. But work with what you have and put out a little extra effort.

Commitment: Park as far away from the door as you can to help towards getting in the recommended 10,000 steps a day.

☐ ☐ ☐ ☐ ☐ ☐ ☐

Journal...

Keep Your Head Up

"All things entail rising and falling timing. You must be able to discern this." – Miyamoto Musashi

To-Do's		Long-Term Goals

This is not a metaphor about keeping your chin up. Your life can be improved by literally keeping your head up. If your chin is up, your eyes are up. If your eyes are up, you can see what's happening around you. If you can see what's happening around you, well...there's no downside to awareness.

You'll also look more confident. **If you are unapologetically taking in everything around you, you'll look like someone who is comfortable with what they see.** If you're shuffling along with your eyes on your toes, well, you know what that looks like. It's not confidence.

You're also less likely to walk in front of a car or a train if you're looking up. And it will force you to pick your feet up when you walk, so that you won't trip over the bumps and cracks in the ground.

Commitment: Keep your head up. Look around. Pay attention. Appear confident.

Journal...

Mix Up Your Rep Schemes

"The less routine the more life." – Amos Branson Alcott

To-Do's		Long-Term Goals

You don't have to look at very many weightlifting articles to learn that you're doing everything completely wrong. Or completely right. You will find the most outlandish contradictions sometimes within the body of the same article. Rep schemes are one of the most common culprits for wild variability.

You will hear that if you want to build muscle, you have to do 8-12 reps of your lifts. For strength, you "never" want to go beyond three reps. **Commit to letting go of the words "always" and "never" when it comes to exercise.** There is much to be said for conventional wisdom, but we are all different, and our ages and goals and injury histories will dictate what works best for each of us.

So, experiment with your rep schemes. If you're keeping a training log you know how many reps you're generally doing.

Commitment: Do more reps. Do fewer. Mix it up and pay attention. Adjust according to your results.

Journal...

Reframing Blame

"When people are lame, they love to blame." – Robert Kiyosaki

To-Do's		Long-Term Goals

Wouldn't it be nice to know that you were blameless for everything? Well, the reality may be closer than you thought. Unfortunately, this doesn't mean you're perfect, or that you're doing everything right. It just means that there is a better way to look at blame, whether you're being blamed, or doing the blaming.

Blaming feels heavy. The word has nothing but negative connotations. But if you start thinking about blame as "responsibility" instead, it takes some of the sting out of it, even if you're the one shouldering the "responsibility" for hurt caused.

It is easier to share responsibility for something than to accept blame. It makes arguments feel like less of a contest, complete with a foe and a victor.

Commitment: The next time you're involved in the blame game, reframe it as responsibility. Agree to share some responsibility. It will make it easier over time.

Journal...

How Much Stuff Do You Need?

"Why the obsession with worldly possessions? When it's your time to go, they have to stay behind, so pack light." – Alex Morritt

To-Do's

✓
✓
✓
✓
✓
✓
✓
✓
✓

This is not a plea for minimalism, although a minimalist lifestyle can make certain things much easier. **This is a reminder that there aren't any truly *logical* reasons as to why buying things should make us happier.** If it does make us happier, this means something. What does it mean? This is a question we each have to answer for ourselves.

But consider that the constant acquisition of stuff is proof of something. Spending money is proof that you make money. Having a new possession might make you feel like a success. After all, how could you buy something if you weren't earning and producing? But how long does that feeling of happiness last for? Not very long in most cases. And often times, attachment to these items will bring a certain amount of discord to your life.

You are already a person worth taking seriously, and loving, and being friends with. So if you get validation from buying things, just ask yourself why.

Commitment: Ask yourself what you get out of your spending habits. Read a book on Buddhism and learn about how it's our attachment to impermanent things that cause us suffering.

Long-Term Goals

☐ ☐ ☐ ☐ ☐ ☐ ☐ ☐ ☐

Journal...

Write An Outline For Your Life

"The more work you put in on your outline and getting the skeleton of your story right, the easier the process is later." – Drew Goodard

To-Do's
✔
✔
✔
✔
✔
✔
✔
✔

Long-Term Goals
☐
☐
☐
☐
☐
☐
☐
☐

Some writers swear by outlines. They plan the story before they start writing it and save themselves a lot of false starts and wasted time. This is how I write. Other writers say that an outline is the bane of existence. That an outline kills spontaneity and, no matter how well you plan, it never looks on paper the way you planned.

Let's leave that behind for a moment and think about what an outline for our lives might look like. It would include the order of events, the themes, essential scenes, major and minor characters, moments of conflict, bottoming out at times, and the climb back up into fulfillment or success or purpose. **If you were assigned to write an outline of your own life, what would it look like?**

To answer this question requires thought and honesty. Give it a try.

Commitment: Pretend you're going to write your story. Outline it. And not just the life you've lived so far, but also the life you've yet to live. Pay special attention to what you leave in, and what you are tempted to leave out.

Journal...

Know The Difference Between Leadership And Management

"If your actions inspire others to dream more, learn more, do more and become more, you are a leader." – John Quincy Adams

To-Do's
✔
✔
✔
✔
✔
✔
✔
✔
✔
✔

Some people are leaders. Some people are managers. Some are both. Some are neither. Some *think* they are one when in fact they are the other. But look at Adams' quote again. I think we all have an idea of someone whom we consider to be a leader. **It is someone who inspires, not just someone who gets people to obey.**

This is one of the major differences between being a leader and a manager. Manager can be a job title, and nothing more. It's just someone who gets paid a manager's salary and is in charge of doing the schedule. Hopefully the manager also has the qualities of a leader, but it's never guaranteed.

A leader makes people *want* to follow. A leader creates an environment or mental space where people can do their best work and do it without being self-conscious. Managers have one primary task, and that is to keep people on task.

Commitment: Strive to be a leader first, and a manager second. Emulate a leader who is admirable to you. You can be a leader in almost any situation—at church, home, school, work, etc…

Long-Term Goals
☐
☐
☐
☐
☐
☐
☐
☐
☐

Journal...

Don't Apologize For What You Like

"There is no such thing as a guilty pleasure." – Douglas Wilson

To-Do's		Long-Term Goals

✔

✔

✔

✔

✔

✔

✔

Do you ever talk about the things you like/love and start with a disclaimer? "I watch _____ but it's just because I need to zone out." "I know it's dumb, but I loved reading____."

There is no reason to apologize or feel guilty about what you like. There's nothing wrong with saying "Good books are the books I like." This might not be an argument that will win over an English professor who assigns you to write a paper on *The Great Gatsby,* but if you're not writing a paper, who cares what anyone else has to say about it?

Don't feel guilty. Or sheepish. You have the right to fill your life and your time with things that make you happy and give you pleasure.

Commitment: The next time you feel the urge to add a disclaimer to something you like, don't. Instead examine, in a deeper sense, why you like that activity.

☐

☐

☐

☐

☐

☐

☐

Journal...

Find The Humor

"Comedy is simply a funny way of being serious." – Peter Ustinov

To-Do's		Long-Term Goals

If you can find something to laugh about, no matter what is happening, you will feel better. Maybe not great, maybe not perfect, but better. And I'm not talking about putting on a chirpy facade and smiling until you actually feel like smiling.

All humor comes from a place of sadness. Or, at the very least, out of an acknowledgement that we wish things were different. We laugh because we're shocked. We laugh because something happened to someone else, and not to us.

We laugh because the alternative is often to cry. Humor is, as Ustinov says, a way of being serious that happens to include laughter. At the very least, if you're looking for the humor in a situation, you're doing something more proactive than wallowing, whether it ultimately succeeds or not.

Commitment: When you are low, find something to laugh about. Anything.

Journal...

Ask Yourself What Happiness Is

"It is not how much we have, but how much we enjoy, that makes happiness." – Charles Spurgeon

To-Do's		Long-Term Goals

Unfortunately, all of us have experienced unhappiness. We know what it means to ask, "Why am I not happy?" But we don't always have a clear definition of what happiness is, besides knowing that it's not *whatever we're feeling when we're unhappy.*

How do you define happiness? **The clearer you can be about it, the better chance you'll have of achieving it.** If happiness means more time with family, then your path is clear. If happiness means a healthier body, then you know how to go about it. But if you just think it's a vague sense of *not this,* then progress may be harder to come by.

Know what happiness is, and go beyond what it is not.

Commitment: Define happiness for yourself. Then take the steps you need to pursue it methodically and single-mindedly. Read *Happier* by Tal Ben-Shahar.

Journal...

Do The Hard Thing First

"A year from now you may wish you had started today." – Karen Lamb

To-Do's
✔
✔
✔
✔
✔
✔

Long-Term Goals
☐
☐
☐
☐
☐
☐

Life can be a joy, or a slog, and everything in between, but there is no escaping this simple reality: **life is an ongoing sequence of tasks and chores.** Some of them will be things you'll look forward to, some are neither worth anticipating or dreading, and some you will flat-out hate.

Doing the things you want to avoid early in your day will set a better tone for the day than putting them last, or putting them off. No one wants to rush towards unpleasantness, but if the unpleasantness is off your to-do list early, it won't be hanging over your head as you go through the day, and you'll be able to enjoy all of the other stuff more.

Commitment: Arrange your daily tasks—those that can be arranged—so that the stuff you're avoiding gets done first. Download the audiobook *Eat That Frog! By Brian Tracy.*

Journal...

August 13

Don't Be Afraid Of Carbs

"I don't believe in the no-carb diet... I have a theory. I think if you give up carbs, you get cranky. You must include them in your daily diet." – Karisma Kapoor

To-Do's

✔

✔

✔

✔

✔

✔

✔

Long-Term Goals

☐

☐

☐

☐

☐

☐

☐

Too many carbs are not good for you. But the same can be said of fats, proteins, water, and vegetables. Anything in excess—true excess—will have a damaging effect if you push it far enough. Carbs get a bad rap for leading to weight and fat gain, and there's some truth to that, if everything else is out of balance and the carbs are excessive.

The truth is, carbs are fuel. If you want energy for your life and your workouts, you need carbs. You don't *only* need carbs. You don't need more grams of carbs than you do protein or fats. But you need carbs. Going without them for too long leads to a state of ketosis. Plus almost every food has carbs. But what you want are complex carbs found in fresh fruits for example, and not simple carbs, like sugary junk foods.

Commitment: Get the right amount of carbs. If you don't have enough energy and you're getting enough sleep, look at carbs first.

Journal...

Be Patient

"Have patience. All things are difficult before they become easy." – Saadi

To-Do's

✔
✔
✔
✔
✔
✔
✔
✔
✔

Long-Term Goals

☐
☐
☐
☐
☐
☐
☐
☐
☐

Life is full of little irritations. The light doesn't turn green fast enough. The line at the grocery store is too long. People talk too loudly. Your boss doesn't understand you. The toast burned. All of these minor nuisances can snowball into one huge bad mood. **And, if left unchecked, bad moods, if they persist long enough, become bad worldviews.**

Patience is the answer. There will always be potential irritations. There's no way to escape this. And the stress that results serves nothing. Wouldn't it be better to just accept that these things will happen, and to work on being patient in the moment?

When you feel the rise of agitation, or your breath gets short, or your face gets hot, just breathe. Tell yourself that it's time to be patient. Carry a book so you can distract yourself when the line gets long. Look around you when you can't make things move faster. Notice things. But breathe and know that it will pass, and that this is not the last time you'll need patience.

Commitment: Be patient. Breathe. Know that there are things that you simply can't rush, and that dwelling on them isn't going to change it. Look up a YouTube video on Mindful Meditation.

Journal...

Attend A Trivia Night

"Why is it trivia? People call it trivia because they know nothing and they are embarrassed about it." – Robbie Coltrane

To-Do's		**Long-Term Goals**

✔

✔

✔

✔

✔

✔

It's fun to know things. It's useful, too. And yet, the hectic pace of adult life often comes at the expense of learning. Sure, we learn the skills required for our jobs, we write our papers in college, but **how often do we simply learn something new for the sheer pleasure of knowing things?**

Trivia nights have gotten really popular at libraries, pubs, and a few other spots. They can be rowdy, but they are a celebration of the fact that there is a lot to know about this world, and it can be a blast to learn.

You'll also meet new people. And if you're cynical about the fact that so many people seem so incurious, a gang of trivia addicts can be a great antidote.

Commitment: Find a trivia night and give it a try.

☐ ☐ ☐ ☐ ☐ ☐

Journal...

Let The Tension Go

"Smile, smile, smile at your mind as often as possible. Your smiling will considerably reduce your mind's tearing tension." – Sri Chimnoy

To-Do's		Long-Term Goals

To-Do's

- ✔
- ✔
- ✔
- ✔
- ✔
- ✔
- ✔
- ✔
- ✔

If you've ever had a massage—and by this point in the book, if you've followed some of the tips, you have!—think about how you feel when it's over. You are feeling the total absence of tension. That's the feeling we're always going for, but **we pick up small tensions throughout the day and store them in our bodies, often without being conscious of them.**

Think about it. Do you notice you're clenching your jaw before it starts hurting? Probably not. Most of us don't make fists from tension and realize "Oh, I just made fists." We only start paying attention when we're aching, or shaking, or can't get our breathing under control.

Learn to pay attention to your body. Do a head-to-toe inventory and note the spots where you are holding tension. Learn to release it. You can always unclench your fists and jaw, lower your shoulders so they're not up by your ears, uncurl your toes, etc. And the more you do it, the less likely these body parts are to return to their contracted state when you're frustrated.

Commitment: Learn where you're holding your tension. Then, learn how to release it.

Long-Term Goals
- ☐
- ☐
- ☐
- ☐
- ☐
- ☐
- ☐
- ☐
- ☐

Journal...

August 17

Keep Healthy Snacks On Hand

"If you get hungry mid-day, a banana is the best snack at your desk, after a workout, or in between classes. Fruit is a very good snack in general." – Marcus Samuelsson

To-Do's		Long-Term Goals

Sometimes things move faster than we plan for, and healthy—or even, consistent—eating can be one of the first casualties when our schedule gets thrown out of whack. But, while it might be hard at times to prepare a healthy meal, there is always enough time to plan for the snacks you'll have on hand.

If you are always carrying a bag of almonds, or raisins, or you've got a banana in your purse or backpack or whatever you use, you'll be ahead of the game. You take a psychological hit when you realize you're hungry and your next meal is hours away. And when you're hungry, you'll be less alert and have less energy.

Commitment: Start carrying snacks with you, the healthier the better. When you first feel hunger, drink water. Wait 10 minutes. Still hungry? Then have some fresh fruit.

Journal...

Define Strength

"Some of us think holding on makes us strong; but sometimes it is letting go." – Herman Hesse

To-Do's

- ✔
- ✔
- ✔
- ✔
- ✔
- ✔
- ✔
- ✔

Long-Term Goals

- ☐
- ☐
- ☐
- ☐
- ☐
- ☐
- ☐
- ☐

Can you think of a test that would prove, conclusively, that one person was stronger than another? We can probably all think of an example that would work for us, but the examples don't hold up to much scrutiny. What is strength? This is the question that must be answered before the test could hold any validity, and this is a question without a clear answer.

Strength means little without context. Is a ballerina stronger than a powerlifter? Yes, at ballet. Is a sprinter stronger than a boxer? Yes, at sprinting. And this doesn't even get into any of the areas of mental and emotional strength.

Once you can define strength, the kind of strength that matters most to you, you can pursue it. It will also allow you to see strength in others in ways you may not have considered.

Commitment: Define strength in the way that is most meaningful to you, then develop it at every chance. Think about emotional and psychological strength too.

Journal...

Consider A Toastmasters Visit

"Speak clearly, if you speak at all; carve every word before you let it fall." – Oliver Wendell Holmes

To-Do's		Long-Term Goals

You've probably heard that the fear of public speaking is second only to the fear of death. What does this mean, that so many people are afraid to get up and say things in front of other people? **How wrong could it actually go?** Where does the fear come from?

Answers will vary from person to person. Do you have a fear of public speaking? Do you know why? If you do, getting over the fear could be worthwhile, even if you have no desires to become a public speaker.

The Toastmasters organization has chapters just about everywhere. Their meetings will be a great way for you to practice speaking and let go of your fears about it.

Commitment: Attend a Toastmasters meeting and see if you like it. If you think it would be helpful to you, consider joining.

Journal...

Don't Give Unsolicited Advice

"You know how advice is. You only want it if it agrees with what you wanted to do anyway." – John Steinbeck

To-Do's		Long-Term Goals

✔

✔

✔

✔

✔

✔

✔

You may be a fount of good advice. This doesn't necessarily mean that everyone is clamoring for it. Not to suggest that you are one, but there are a lot of well-meaning busybodies whose insistence at giving advice to everyone, in every situation, turn people off to the point where **the message gets lost.**

If you're in the habit of offering advice, consider taking a break, even if it's just to see how often you give advice. So many of the things we know we should be doing come down to common sense, and it's hard not to feel patronized when someone holds forth on something you're totally aware of already.

Commitment: Don't give advice unless asked. When asked, be generous, but don't pretend you know things you don't just so you can feel like wise old Socrates. Just speak from your own personal experiences.

☐ ☐ ☐ ☐ ☐ ☐ ☐

Journal...

Pick Up The Check Sometimes

"Let us try to teach generosity and altruism, because we are born selfish." – Richard Dawkins

To-Do's

✔

✔

✔

✔

✔

Going out to eat with friends or family can be a blast. For some people it takes on the quality of a ritual. And most of the time, when it's time to pay, the check gets split however many ways it needs to.

Do you ever pick up the check? There would be times when the cost would be prohibitive, but there are probably also times when you could afford it. The good will this creates, and the pleasure you can get out of an act of spontaneous generosity, can work wonders to defray the expense.

Few things are as memorable as a generous person.

Commitment: Pick up the check sometime in the next month.

Long-Term Goals

☐

☐

☐

☐

☐

Journal...

Don't Inflate Your Achievements

"If I weren't too proud, I'd boast of my exaggerated opinion of myself." – Bauvard

To-Do's

Long-Term Goals

You are a person who has done things worth being of, and who will do more in the future, even if you don't know it or can't admit it. But there's never going to be a reason for bragging or boasting. **Being proud of our achievements is different than using them for validation and applause.**

And that's the thing with overinflating our achievements. It's obvious when it happens, and it obviously means we need something out of telling people out of our achievements. And if you tell someone about something you've done, and they don't swoon or clap, maybe you have the temptation to make it just a little bigger. A little more impressive.

Don't do it. There's no reason to lie.

Commitment: Don't inflate your achievements. Instead, think of yourself as a work-in-progress, think of the becoming, the things you're going to accomplish...

Journal...

Don't Beg People To Let You Help Them

"There is no exercise better for the heart than reaching down and lifting people up." – John Holmes

To-Do's

- ✔
- ✔
- ✔
- ✔
- ✔
- ✔
- ✔

Long-Term Goals

- ☐
- ☐
- ☐
- ☐
- ☐
- ☐
- ☐

You may have had a critical time in your life where another person helped you turn it around. Or maybe someone even saved you—from circumstances, from yourself, from a skewed perspective or unproductive way of thinking. And there will be times when you can do the same for others.

While we should help the people who we can help, there is a point where a person must take responsibility for their own well being. **People can become infatuated with, and habituated to, their own melancholy, loneliness, and suffering.** When people proclaim that they want happiness, but refuse to change their own actions (think of this as a form of negativity,) do not beg them, over and over, to listen to reason or to accept your help.

Sometimes you can't fix it. Sometimes real change has to come from inside someone.

Commitment: Don't beg people to let you help them. We are all responsible for our own lives, even those we love the most who are lost.

Journal...

Practice The Same Lift Every Day For A Month

"Practice does not make perfect. Only perfect practice makes perfect." – Vince Lombardi

To-Do's		Long-Term Goals

If you want to learn how to do something, frequent practice helps. No one plays piano scales once a month and expects to become a master pianist. It's the same with practicing lifts in the weight room, with a couple of caveats. You can't go into the gym every day for a month and squat, for example, with maximum effort. That would tax your system to the point where it would simply be a gut check with a heavy cost, not productive practice.

But if you went in every day for a month and just practiced the movement, you would see improvement in your technique and strength and confidence. Making it every day for a month could mean doing less weight, fewer sets, fewer reps per set, etc. **You'd want to tweak it however you needed to in order to *practice*, not to grind through it.**

And a month is an arbitrary period. If you want to improve at a lift, increasing the frequency of practice will help you.

Commitment: Pick a lift you want to improve at and find a way to practice it every day for a month. Focus on form, not weight, strength, or power. Note your results.

Journal...

Pay Down Your Credit Card Debt

"You can't be in debt and win. It doesn't work." – Dave Ramsey

To-Do's		Long-Term Goals

✔

✔

✔

✔

✔

✔

If you're in credit card debt, you have to earn money to pay it off. If you're going to earn money, you have to sell your labor, time, and/or skills. Time you spend working to pay off debt is time spent on someone else's behalf. **Think about this: if you are working to get out of credit card debt, you are working for someone else.**

Credit card debt can be a nuisance, or it can get out of hand and turn into a taskmaster that dictates your schedule, how many hours you work, how much time you can afford to take off, and what you can buy for yourself. Credit card debt limits your choices. Credit card debt is pure stress.

Commitment: If you have a lot of credit card debt, see a financial planner and come up with a strategy to end it. Consider cutting up your credit cards, except for one.

☐
☐
☐
☐
☐
☐

Journal...

Limit Your Internet Information Intake

"Getting information off the Internet is like taking a drink from a fire hydrant." – Mitchell Kapor

To-Do's		Long-Term Goals

We have more access to more information than ever before. Today, this is truer than it was yesterday. It will be truer tomorrow than it is today. And the ocean of accessible information now makes it possible to feel like we are learning, when in fact it is possible that we are simply browsing more information.

Consuming information quickly and constantly sounds great, unless none of it gets absorbed in a way that is useful. Scanning ten articles about the Civil War on the Internet may do less for us than carefully and thoughtfully reading one book about it.

Commitment: This week, limit your internet information intake by half. And when you decide to read something, *really* read it, don't just scan. Take notes on what you read.

Journal...

Focus On One Task At A Time

"Many people feel they must multi-task because everybody else is multitasking, but this is partly because they are all interrupting each other so much." – Marilyn vos Savant

To-Do's		Long-Term Goals

The fact that we can multitask has nothing to do with whether we should. There's no disputing that it's better to do things well than to do them less well, and yet, the gospel of multitasking continues to grow. Truth is, there is no such thing as "multitasking." We are actually "switching" attention between two tasks.

Make a tally of the tasks you must do in a normal day. Now be honest: how many of them need to overlap? Of course there are exceptions. If your boss demands that you respond to an email or make a call while you're occupied with something else, you should probably listen.

But most things can be laid out in sequence, with complete attention given to each one. There's no reason not to. You'll wind up saving time and doing everything better.

Commitment: Try it and see. Take a break from multitasking for a few days. When you think you're multitasking, see it for what it really is, switching.

Journal...

Be Willing To Lose An Argument

"Silence is one of the hardest arguments to refute." – Josh Billings

To-Do's		Long-Term Goals

We don't always have to be right, and yet, it is possible to go on proclaiming how right we are, even *after* we know that we're wrong. This is different than the tip on not having to have the last word. **This is a suggestion that sometimes it is okay just to let the other person be right, even if they're wrong.**

There are arguments that you can let go. This doesn't mean that if someone is proudly saying, "Racism is wonderful!" that you must let that person be right just not to make waves. They might not be worth arguing with, but you don't have to let something go which you find abhorrent.

But how many arguments have real stakes, or high implications for our morals? Having peace is much more important than being right.

Commitment: The next time you're in an argument, if you can, ask yourself if you could live with losing. If so, if it will spare both of you emotional turmoil, consider just letting it go.

Journal...

Make Time To Be Lazy

"Rest and be thankful." – William Wordsworth

To-Do's	
✔	
✔	
✔	
✔	
✔	
✔	
✔	
✔	

Long-Term Goals

☐ ☐ ☐ ☐ ☐ ☐ ☐ ☐

When you get a day off, do you really give yourself a day off? Or do you spend it catching up on chores, running errands, or even continuing the work you should have left at your workplace? You're certainly not alone.

Days of rest are often anything but. They are days to play catch up. **If you take a day off and you're not rejuvenated by the end of it, you could have done it better.** If you're busy, or you have a hard time not bringing work home with you, this can be tough. But maybe not as tough as *never taking a real break*.

If you have a day off, you *must* make it feel like a day off in some way. Take a nap. Channel surf. Read. Something just for you. Turn off your phone. Your brain will thank you, and so will your energy. And when you go back to work, you'll be better for it.

Commitment: Make your days off resemble something like days off. Do something you love but haven't done in awhile, like paint, practice guitar, or hike.

Journal...

_____
_____
_____
_____
_____
_____
_____
_____
_____
_____
_____
_____
_____
_____
_____
_____
_____
_____
_____
_____
_____

Embrace Aging

"Aging has a wonderful beauty and we should have respect for that." – Eartha Kitt

To-Do's		Long-Term Goals

To-Do's

- ✓
- ✓
- ✓
- ✓
- ✓
- ✓
- ✓
- ✓
- ✓

Long-Term Goals

- ☐
- ☐
- ☐
- ☐
- ☐
- ☐
- ☐
- ☐
- ☐

We don't have to like aging, but we can't fight it forever. It happens every day, and every moment. But we can (and should) accept it. There is no more denying the aging process, outside of maintaining healthy bodies and nutritional habits, than there is holding back the ocean.

Often, when I hear people wishing they were younger, they're talking about their younger bodies, or for times in which they had less physical pain or more physical strength. This is understandable and poignant. But I don't hear very many people wish they could regain the callowness and naiveté that accompanies youth. No one seems to want to relieve the melodramatic storms of high school.

No one longs for a return to immaturity and a diminished degree of wisdom. If you can't seem to avoid mourning the loss of your youth, at least find a way to acknowledge the benefits of greater maturity, wisdom, and, self-knowledge, and autonomy that are the rewards of age.

Commitment: Come up with ten advantages that come with aging. Refer to them every time you find yourself wishing you were younger.

Journal...

If All Else Fails

"You'll reach into your wallet to brandish a photograph of a new puppy, and a friend will say, 'Oh, no - not pictures.'" – Caroline Knapp

To-Do's
✔
✔
✔
✔
✔
✔
✔
✔
✔

Long-Term Goals

☐
☐
☐
☐
☐
☐
☐
☐
☐

Now, I know that not everyone is an animal lover, but people who say they don't like animals are usually thinking about *living* with animals. Just about anyone can look at a kitten and think that it's adorable. Whether or not they want to take it home and care for it is irrelevant to this entry.

Sometimes nothing feels like it helps. Nothing cheers us up. For all the skepticism I express in this book about certain aspects of the internet, it is absolutely the pinnacle of at least one thing: **cute animal pictures.**

So I'm suggesting, with a mostly straight face, that if you just can't find anything to be glad about...go to a computer, type in "cute animal pictures," and give yourself a few minutes to scroll through them. It might not help, but sometimes it might be the only thing that will. In any event, it is a very, very easy experiment to try.

Commitment: When you're out of last resorts, resort to this one—look at some pictures of cute animals, baby ones, preferably. See if it helps. It might give you the tiniest nudge back in the right direction.

Journal...

September

Learn Some Basic Anatomy

"Whoever named it necking was a poor judge of anatomy." – Groucho Marx

To-Do's

✔

✔

✔

✔

✔

✔

✔

Long-Term Goals

☐

☐

☐

☐

☐

☐

☐

Chances are, at some point you'll be sitting in front of a doctor who will want to know how you're feeling, when your symptoms started, and for you to describe anything you can about the source and location of the discomfort. This is when you may find out that you don't know much about the body. After all, most of us aren't doctors, right?

Learning some basic anatomy will teach you how to pay better attention to what is happening in your body. Not to mention that anatomy is simply a fascinating subject. If you're not opposed to dark humor and morbid subject matter, Mary Roach's book *Stiff: The Curious Lives of Human Cadavers* will show you just how fascinating your body is, from its first cell...to its very last.

Commitment: Learn some basic anatomy. There are some wonderful, inexpensive flash cards that can help you make great progress with brief, daily sessions.

Journal...

Should You Care What People Think?

"You'll worry less about what people think about you when you realize how seldom they do." – David Foster Wallace

To-Do's

- ✔
- ✔
- ✔
- ✔
- ✔
- ✔
- ✔
- ✔

Long-Term Goals

- ☐
- ☐
- ☐
- ☐
- ☐
- ☐
- ☐
- ☐

"I don't care what anyone thinks about me," is the rallying cry of the insecure, melodramatic teenager. And of course, when a teenager says it, what they're really saying is that they care *desperately* what people think about them. This can be a highwire act as adults: you should not let what other people think of you limit your ambitions or hinder your confidence. And yet, there may be times when you need to care what other people think of you.

If your boss thinks you're lazy, you should care if keeping your job is important. If your spouse thinks that you're being distant, you should care if keeping your spouse is important to you. But most of the time, worrying about what other people think does not do anything but wear you out. **They're not aware that you're stewing about what they think about you.**

Commitment: The next time you're worrying about what people think of you, just ask yourself if it really matters. And if they were thinking something about you that was unfair, your being aware of it doesn't change their thoughts anyway.

Journal...

Where Do You Get Your News?

"Good news is rare these days, and every glittering ounce of it should be cherished and hoarded and worshipped and fondled like a priceless diamond." – Hunter S. Thompson

To-Do's
✔
✔
✔
✔
✔
✔
✔
✔

The Internet, with its near-bottomless masses of blogs, social media, digital extensions of traditional news media, and more, has made it easier to stay up to date as far as the news goes. However, the fact that everyone can now report on what's happening, in real time, and that people all over the world can see it, requires accuracy and judgment in order to make it worthwhile.

The truth is, news worth reading is often news worth paying for. Heading to Twitter to watch as an incident unfolds can be enlightening, if the facts being reported are accurate. But for an actual analysis of the event, we would do well to give it a couple of days before reading about it in a respected publication. This does not discount the importance of citizen journalism. But websites are in the business of getting clicks. It is better to be saying something *wrong* than to be saying nothing at all, when a website's competitors are all reporting. **And this *will* affect your world view.**

Commitment: Choose a couple of news sources that you trust. Cut others out.

Long-Term Goals
- ☐
- ☐
- ☐
- ☐
- ☐
- ☐
- ☐
- ☐

Journal...

_____
_____
_____
_____
_____
_____
_____
_____
_____
_____
_____
_____
_____
_____
_____
_____
_____
_____
_____
_____
_____

Forget About Miracle Diets

"Fads are the kiss of death. When the fad goes away, you go with it." – Conway Twitty

To-Do's		Long-Term Goals
✔		☐
✔		☐
✔		☐
✔		☐
✔		☐
✔		☐
✔		☐
✔		☐

You can dress it up any way you want, but fat loss and weight loss are not complicated. Now, the emotional and mental issues surrounding stress eating and comfort eating and trickier, but let's talk about the simple fact of weight loss.

If you consume fewer calories than you expend—putting yourself in a caloric deficit—you will lose weight. This is still the reality behind the Atkins Diet, the Paleo Diet, South Beach, juice fasts, and on and on and on. They go about the same thing in different ways and they espouse differing philosophies, but those are largely frameworks that underlie the same truth—**eat healthy food, and eat fewer calories to lose weight and fat.**

The promise of a miracle, or a shortcut, is tempting. Who wouldn't want to believe it? But if you think you can have the body of your dreams in a month, you'll be discouraged when a month goes by and the hype didn't live up to the reality.

Commitment: Forget the miracles. Eat healthy. Love your current body so much that you wish to improve it.

Journal...

_____
_____
_____
_____
_____
_____
_____
_____
_____
_____
_____
_____
_____
_____
_____
_____
_____
_____
_____
_____

Learn To Read The Labels

"Once you learn the basic rules of good nutrition, you'll realize it's not so complicated. It doesn't matter if you're running errands or 13 miles, you need enough fuel to last all day. Proper nutrition is the difference between feeling exhausted and getting the most out of a workout." – Summer Sanders

To-Do's		Long-Term Goals
✔	If you go to a grocery store and watch people putting things in their cart, you probably won't see very many people reading the labels. Now, maybe this is because they've already done it and they already know what they're dealing with. **More likely is that they don't read the labels because, well, it's easier not to.**	☐
✔		☐
✔	But even if you do read the labels, it's worth knowing how they work. The ingredient that comprises the largest chunk of the product is listed first. At a glance, you can also see how many calories per serving, the serving size, protein in grams, fats, carbs, and more.	☐
✔		☐
✔		☐
✔	It sounds like a lot, and it would be, if you were obsessive about it. But like anything, the more you practice reading the labels, the more you'll be able to take in at a glance. And you'll give yourself more chances at healthy eating and living.	☐
✔		☐
✔	**Commitment:** Learn to read the labels. It's an easy habit once you commit to it. Make sure you are aware of the serving size and number of servings per container, then multiply accordingly.	☐

Journal...

_____
_____
_____
_____
_____
_____
_____
_____
_____
_____
_____
_____
_____
_____
_____
_____
_____
_____
_____
_____

Sleep With A Pillow Under Or Between Your Knees

"Sleep is that golden chain that ties health and our bodies together." – Thomas Dekker

To-Do's

- ✔
- ✔
- ✔
- ✔
- ✔

Because we spend so much time sleeping, it is worth doing it right. **Right, in this case, means waking up without pain that sets in during the night.** Even if you have the right bed, sleeping in less than optimal positions for the spine can cause lingering discomfort that follows you into your day.

One of the easiest experiments to try is to sleep with a pillow under your knees, if you're a back sleeper. If you sleep on your side, try putting the pillow between your knees. This can sometimes align the spin in a better position, and you'll feel better in the morning.

Commitment: Try sleeping with a pillow under or between your knees. See if you feel differently the next morning.

Long-Term Goals

- ☐
- ☐
- ☐
- ☐
- ☐

Journal...

Be Approachable

"To combat social awkwardness, I would just act like I couldn't be bothered - that kind of aloof persona or aloof demeanor. It's so off-putting." – Janeane Garofalo

To-Do's		Long-Term Goals

Think of someone who you consider approachable. What is it that you are picturing? Is he or she scowling or is the face relaxed? What's the posture like? Are they squinting furiously, typing at full speed, walking with such purpose and haste that it's as if they are on their way to meet with destiny itself?

There will be times when you don't want people to come up and talk to you. It stinks to be interrupted while working or trying to get a task done, just because someone knows that you're nice and will listen.

But if you can project an aura of approachability, you will probably feel better inside. **To be approachable, even if you're alone, is to project calm, good humor, and an absence of tension.**

Commitment: Take time out of each hour to check in with yourself. Are you being approachable? What could you do differently? Do you feel inner peace?

Journal...

Make An Honest Inventory Of Your Biases

"Two quite opposite qualities equally bias our minds - habits and novelty." – Jean de la Bruyere

To-Do's		Long-Term Goals

From the dictionary:

✔

Bias—prejudice in favor of or against one thing, person, or group compared with another, usually in a way considered to be unfair.

✔

One of the most uncomfortable experiences you can go through is to make an honest assessment or your own biases and prejudices. **We all have them, whether consciously or subconsciously, and pretending we don't is naive.** Sit down and really try to do this. You don't have to tell anyone or announce your results.

✔

✔

✔

Sit down and think about all of the people, groups, ideas, and experiences that were your upbringing. Which of them do you feel have the greatest potential to have shaped your worldview? Especially the negative and unfounded ones. Which areas are you less likely to be open-minded in? Do you have any biases solely based on stereotypes?

✔

✔

This is not a chance to indict yourself for anything. It is just a thought experiment that can benefit you greatly, if you can be honest enough to do it thoroughly.

✔

Commitment: Take a bias inventory. Think about the implications. Change what you can change.

Journal...

Your Life Is Not Big Enough To Hate

"This is what I'm saying; you hate your life. But you don't know what life is. Life is too huge for you to possibly hate. If you hate life, you haven't seen enough of it. If you hate your life, it's because your life is too small and doesn't fit you. However big you think your life is, it's nothing compared to what's out there." – Augusten Burroughs

To-Do's		Long-Term Goals

We will all have times when, if we do not hate our lives, that we may at the very least be weary of them. But to say "I hate my life," is to act like you know more than you do. The Burrough's quote above says it so well that I don't want to belabor the point.

There are always ways to expand your horizons. There are always ways to look at things with a new perspective. Whether we choose those options during our lowest points is up to us.

When you are up against the wall and you are tired of everything you know, it is time to do or see or learn or feel something else. And there is always a way. You don't have to take it, but you can't deny that it is true.

Commitment: The next time you think you hate your life, refer to the Burrough's quote at the top of this entry. Think about what you can do to make your life bigger. Do something that scares you.

Journal...

Don't Interrupt

"And now, excuse me while I interrupt myself." – Murray Walker

To-Do's

- ✔
- ✔
- ✔
- ✔
- ✔
- ✔
- ✔

Long-Term Goals

- ☐
- ☐
- ☐
- ☐
- ☐
- ☐
- ☐

We all know what it feels like to be interrupted. Therefore, you probably don't want to be seen as someone who interrupts others. There's a natural give and take in most conversations, and there are natural times to interject something to add to a conversation. **But real, discourteous interruption is something to avoid.**

It shows that the interrupter is self-centered and a poor listener. To interrupt someone is essentially to say, "That reminds me of something more interesting and now I'm going to say it!"

I've known a lot of people who everyone thought were fascinating conversationalists. The ironic thing was, those people were the ones who let other people do most of the talking.

Commitment: Don't interrupt others. You'll get your turn. And when you do, make sure it's worth speaking.

Journal...

Remember the Sacrifices Of Others

"There is no decision that we can make that doesn't come with some sort of balance or sacrifice." – Simon Sinek

To-Do's

✔

✔

✔

✔

✔

✔

✔

Long-Term Goals

☐

☐

☐

☐

☐

☐

☐

So many of the good things we have are possible because of the sacrifices of others. It could be our parents, who took the time and spared no expense in raising us properly and making sure we had what we needed. It could be the leaders who formed the countries in which we live, who had the foresight to ensure that we would be free down the road.

Our friends sacrifice for us, as we do for them. And the list goes on. **No one can achieve as much as possible without the contributions of others, and to be in any sort of relationship with others is to sacrifice.** We will always be in a better position to receive, if we're always conscientious enough to give our talents and efforts to others when they need them.

Commitment: Give credit to the sacrifice of others. Be grateful. Relationships by definition are sacrifices.

Journal...

Forget About What's Fair

"Life is unfair. I got nothing but the best." – Jean Marais

To-Do's

- ✔
- ✔
- ✔
- ✔
- ✔
- ✔
- ✔
- ✔

Long-Term Goals

- ☐
- ☐
- ☐
- ☐
- ☐
- ☐
- ☐
- ☐

Life is not fair. This is a fact. No matter how well we might bear our burdens, it is not fair that some of us will get cancer, people will get hit by cars, airplanes will crash because of mechanical failure, our bodies will age and devolve. Our minds are susceptible to the cruelties of dementia, and human cruelty runs rampant in too much of the world.

Acknowledging that life is unfair can be a liberating act, as it can lead to the question, "Who promised me fairness?" Or, "Why should things be fair for me when they're brutally unjust for so many others?"

The unfairness of life can have a galvanizing effect. **It can urge us to make the most of our time, knowing that our futures may be as uncertain as anyone else's.** Few things encourage us to use our time as productively as the realization that our time here on earth is tenuous and precious.

Commitment: Forget about what's fair. Instead, ask yourself what you can do to improve or change your current situation.

Journal...

September 13

Don't Give Up Too Much Control

"Only you can control your future." – Dr. Seuss

To-Do's

- ✔
- ✔
- ✔
- ✔
- ✔
- ✔
- ✔

To be in a relationship—whether it's a relationship with family, coworkers, or a significant other—is to give up some control. You will be required to make decisions whose outcomes do not only affect just you. But this does not mean that you have to give up all control.

It is always important to know that you have a choice. Yes, you have responsibilities to others, but those responsibilities do not have to be the factor that makes all of your decisions for you.

The surest way to know if you've given up too much control is to make a list of the things you do just for yourself. If you can't come up with anything, you are not prioritizing your own well-being, and your loved ones would want you to be taking time for yourself, as well as for them.

Commitment: Ask yourself why you made the decisions you did today. Were they for yourself? For others? Could it have been another way? Make a list of the things you do solely for yourself.

Long-Term Goals

- ☐
- ☐
- ☐
- ☐
- ☐
- ☐
- ☐

Journal...

September 14

If You Want To Grow, Rest

"You don't grow in the gym." – Stan Efferding

To-Do's	Long-Term Goals

✔

✔

✔

✔

✔

✔

✔

Not everyone wants to get bigger muscles, but greater strength is a benefit to everyone, so if you're not a bodybuilder, feel free to view this tip through the lens of growing your strength. When you're gung-ho at the beginning of a program, it can be tempting to want to go every day and spend more time than necessary in the gym.

This can be counterproductive. Your muscles can't grow without rest, and your nervous system has to recover as well. **Going to the gym constantly will make you leaner, but it will take away more than it gives you.**

If you want to grow, you have to eat a lot, lift weights that are heavy for you, and sleep a lot. It can be hard to show the restraint it takes to stay out of the gym if you're a fitness addict, but it's the only way to muscle growth.

Commitment: If your goals require you to go to the gym less often, then cut back.

☐ ☐ ☐ ☐ ☐ ☐ ☐

Journal...

September 15

Take Pride Of Ownership (In Yourself)

"Show class, have pride, and display character. If you do, winning takes care of itself." – Paul Bryant

To-Do's

- ✔
- ✔
- ✔
- ✔
- ✔
- ✔
- ✔

Long-Term Goals

- ☐
- ☐
- ☐
- ☐
- ☐
- ☐
- ☐

You probably wouldn't buy a nice car and immediately start ignoring its maintenance. And you probably wouldn't buy a bunch of food and drinks and spill them all over it, and then ignore the stains. This would be true with just about any expensive possession we could own. We take care of the things that we are proud to own.

But what about ourselves? Our bodies? Our minds? **If someone observed your habits for a week, would they conclude that you take pride of ownership in yourself?** Would they see you nurturing your mind and fortifying your body and health? If not, it says something about your priorities. Some people take better care of their cars than they do themselves, which is a sad statement.

Commitment: Pretend that you're being watched. Show the observer that you have enough pride in yourself so that they could not reach any other conclusion. Start by dressing nicely today.

Journal...

Write Your Own Ideal Obituary

"Defeat the fear of death and you welcome the death of fear." – G. Gordon Liddy

To-Do's		Long-Term Goals

This might sound morbid, but it's all about perspective. We all know that we will die. **An obituary is, in its way, a celebration of the life lived.** It is a summation of experience and loved ones and of the passions and interests and contributions of the deceased.

How would you need to live in order for someone to write your ideal obituary? What would you have to do? How would you need to treat people? What passions would you have to pursue? What would you most want people to say about you after you died?

An obituary can be a map to what's important to you. At the very least, it will force you to think about the kind of life you want to live. Live your life in a way so that your obituary will be longer than a paragraph.

Commitment: Write your obituary. Live in a way that will make it true.

Journal...

Make The Exercise Matter

"You don't get any medal for trying something, you get medals for results." – Bill Parcells

To-Do's		Long-Term Goals

Observe a handful of people at the gym and you will see at least a couple of them that seem to be in a great hurry. I don't mean people doing circuits or cardio work that requires them to move quickly. I just mean people who look like they just want to get *done.* They're probably the people counting reps and ignoring technique, so that they can check the box that says *I went to the gym today.*

It is admirable that they cared enough to go and get a workout. **But results must be the focus, not just the time put in.** This is true for all areas of life. When you do an exercise, you should be striving to make the set *matter,* not to make it *end* by racing through it. Take the time to pay attention, to feel the working muscle, to move smoothly and with confidence, and to get the results out of the movement that you deserve, since you cared enough to go to the gym.

Commitment: Don't rush in the gym. Lift thoughtfully and with concentration. Don't rush through life. Make decisions deliberately and with purpose.

Journal...

Just Put Your Shoes On

"Once something is a passion, the motivation is there." – Michael Schumacher

To-Do's

- ✔
- ✔
- ✔
- ✔
- ✔
- ✔
- ✔
- ✔

Long-Term Goals

- ☐
- ☐
- ☐
- ☐
- ☐
- ☐
- ☐
- ☐

I heard a story once about a woman who said she never had any trouble getting to the gym, as long as she just put her shoes on. For her, putting her shoes on was the hardest part of it all. If she could just make herself lace up those sneakers, there was no way she wasn't going to the gym. But it was easy to ignore the shoes, to not put them on, and, well, if she didn't have shoes on, she couldn't very well go to the gym, could she?

We all have an equivalent of putting those shoes on. There's a point at which, if we can each just get past it, the rest of the course is set. If you're a writer, it might be sharpening a pencil or sitting down at your desk. If you're a painter who procrastinates, it could be mixing your paint. If you're always late paying your bills, then it could be just setting up automatic bank payments.

Commitment: Know what your sticking point is, and focus on that. Don't think about getting to the gym—or whatever your equivalent is—think about getting your shoes on.

Journal...

How Are We The Same? How Are We Different?

"The purpose of anthropology is to make the world safe for human differences." – Ruth Benedict

To-Do's

- ✔
- ✔
- ✔
- ✔
- ✔
- ✔
- ✔

Long-Term Goals

- ☐
- ☐
- ☐
- ☐
- ☐
- ☐
- ☐

Imagine that an alien research team descended and selected ten people for an object lesson. The ten people were the ten most different people on the globe. The aliens then challenge the rest of humanity to a test: explain to us how these ten people are the same.

If you spend much time paying attention, even if you feel like no one understands you, you will see that we are all the same on many levels. Once we see that others are like us, it not only makes it easier to understand them, it opens the door to the possibility that maybe we're not as hard to understand, as isolated, as we might think.

This is the key to true empathy and love. **The ability to recognize yourself in others, and them in you.**

Commitment: This week, with every person you interact with, think briefly about how each of you are similar, and how you are different. Soon you will see that we have more in common than not.

Journal...

Use Your Non-Dominant Hand

"I'd give my right arm to be ambidextrous." – Yogi Berra

To-Do's

- ✔
- ✔
- ✔
- ✔
- ✔
- ✔
- ✔
- ✔
- ✔

Long-Term Goals

- ☐
- ☐
- ☐
- ☐
- ☐
- ☐
- ☐
- ☐
- ☐

Even though you probably get along just fine with your dominant hand, think about how much easier certain things could be if you could use either hand just as well. It's hard to picture a downside. And yet, even though you may never reach total interchangeability with your hands, there are a lot of ways to slowly bring up your skill with your non-dominant hand.

You start by simply doing *more* things than usual with that hand. If you're right handed, try brushing your teeth with your left. Or reaching to take a book off a shelf. Or turning that book's pages. Once you get more confident, practice writing, or throwing. It's fun to see how quick the progress can be, and down the road, it's useful.

There is such vast interplay between the hemispheres of the brain and the sides of the body that they each control, that it's hard to imagine that, at some level, developing the non-dominant side of the body might not have some impact on our very brains.

Commitment: Use your non-dominant hand more often. Focus on the areas that feel the clumsiest. They'll have the biggest payoff.

Journal...

Take Off Your Watch When You Can

"Don't watch the clock; do what it does. Keep going." – Sam Levenson

To-Do's
✔
✔
✔
✔
✔
✔

Time goes by and there's nothing we can do about it. The world ages and so do we. **But time—as in, hours, minutes, weeks, and *work-weeks*—are completely manmade constructs.** This kind of time is the stuff of timesheets, punching a clock, being in meetings at the right time, etc.

On your off days, when you don't need to wear a watch—or look at the clock on your phone—consider ditching it. If you don't actually *need* to know what time it is, it's almost impossible to feel rushed, as long as you aren't checking a clock. It can free your mind up and tell it not to hurry, that it doesn't matter if you go at a leisurely pace, and that you are free to direct your attention where you like.

Commitment: When you can, lose the watch. Enjoy the time you have instead of counting it down.

Long-Term Goals
☐
☐
☐
☐
☐
☐

Journal...

You Are A Scientist

"Science is a way of thinking much more than it is a body of knowledge." – Carl Sagan

To-Do's		Long-Term Goals

As Dr. Siddartha Mukherjeed says in his book *The Emperor of All Maladies: A Biography of Cancer,* "Science begins with counting." So much of the book you're reading has to do with improving our ability to pay attention. Why? So that we can track our progress and so make ever greater progress. And all along the way, we are counting.

A scientist is results-oriented. A scientist asks questions and seeks to find answers. The answers generally lead to more questions. **Life is a constant game of reevaluating and changing course based on the questions we ask and the results we see.**

As Sagan says, science is a way of thinking. It is the way of thinking that leads to personal progress. And it is the personal progress of individuals that eventually leads to progress for humankind as a whole.

Commitment: Think like a scientist. How? Evaluate. Think. Focus on results. Course correct.

Journal...

Question Causation

"Fate is the endless chain of causation, whereby things are; the reason or formula by which the world goes on."
– Citium Zeno

✔

✔

✔

✔

✔

✔

✔

✔

✔

☐

☐

☐

☐

☐

☐

☐

☐

☐

It is better to ask "What?" than "Why?" Here's what I mean. When we ask "Why did this happen?" whether it's a sprained ankle, a dip in the stock market, an illness, or an unfair change of events, we are assuming that there is a concrete answer. This is rarely the case. Scientists do not talk about what they know. They talk about the probability of event A causing event B.

Now, suppose you hit your hand with a hammer. We "know" why your hand hurts, right. But a scientist might still say something like, "There is a 99.999999% probability that event A (the hammer hitting the hand) caused event B (the pain)." It leaves the door open to other alternatives, and this is the key to open-mindedness and progression.

So, if we're jettisoning "Why?" what good does it do to replace it with "What?" Consider this: if you ask "What?" As in, "What just happened?" **You're simply looking at a chain of events, knowing you might be wrong.** Ask "What happened, what happened before that, and what happened after?" Then you can rearrange the sequence for different results next time, possibly.

Commitment: The next time you're tempted to ask "Why?" ask "What?" instead. Think of life as a sequence of events.

Journal...

Stopping. Starting. Keeping On.

"I think it's very important to have a feedback loop, where you're constantly thinking about what you've done and how you could be doing it better." – Elon Musk

To-Do's
✔
✔
✔
✔
✔
✔
✔

Long-Term Goals

☐
☐
☐
☐
☐
☐

What should we stop doing? What should we start doing? What should we keep doing? These three questions, asked together and answered thoughtfully, would solve the problems of just about every Human Resources department in the world.

But these three questions could benefit anyone, at any point in their lives. Try it. What should I stop doing? Like wasting every Sunday, watching football. What should I keep doing? Like waking up an hour earlier to work on my book. What should I start doing? Like incorporating green smoothies for breakfast. If you have goals, you will not have any problem answering these questions. It's a simple, effective exercise that can help you attain your goals or get you back on track.

Commitment: Ask and answer these three questions regularly. Weekly, at a minimum. Daily is ideal. Adjust your actions based on your answers.

Journal...

Give People The Benefit Of The Doubt

"I give everyone the benefit of the doubt." – Claudia Christian

To-Do's
✔
✔
✔
✔
✔
✔
✔

Long-Term Goals

- ☐
- ☐
- ☐
- ☐
- ☐
- ☐
- ☐

If someone has ever betrayed your trust, it can be hard to let them into your confidence again. If multiple people betray your trust over time, you can get sour on the whole of humanity. **And if *you* ever betray someone else's trust, you'll understand that anyone is capable of doing it.**

And yet, we will be healthier, mentally, and more optimistic if we give people the benefit of the doubt. It doesn't feel good, even when it feels justified, to make up our minds about people before they get a chance to make their own impressions.

However, this does not mean that you have to give people unlimited chances. There's a point where it's probably no longer healthy for you to give people the benefit of the doubt *again.* Be thoughtful, take it case by case, and do what is best for *you.*

Commitment: Give people the benefit of the doubt until there's a reason not to.

Journal...

Practice Isometrics

"I do isometrics in church so while I'm doing my soul some good, I'm doing my body some good, too." – Grace Kelly

To-Do's		Long-Term Goals

✔

✔

✔

✔

✔

✔

✔

Isometrics might be the simplest form of exercise or strength training that there is. You push or pull on an immovable object. If you put your shoulder against your house and strained as if you were trying to scoot it across the room, that's an isometric exercise. Bruce Lee claimed that he would do isometrics at red lights, taking the chance to press against the roof of his vehicle for a few seconds.

All weight training and strength training involve the contraction of muscles. You can generate a contraction with a dumbbell, kettlebell, or isometrics. The nice thing about isometrics is that you can do them anywhere. Push on the earth. Push on a wall. Pull on the railing that leads down the steps at work. Anything can work.

Commitment: If you're looking for ways to sneak in a little extra strength training, try isometrics. Find multiple times and situations during the day where you can push or pull on an immovable object.

☐
☐
☐
☐
☐
☐
☐

Journal...

Try The Pomodoro Technique

"Perfectionism prevents action. Waiting until you have devised the perfect solution to something is merely a form of procrastination." – Staffan Noteberg

To-Do's

✔
✔
✔
✔
✔
✔
✔
✔
✔

Francesco Cirillo developed the Pomodoro Technique as an experiment to see whether frequent breaks during a workday or a work project could result in greater results and better mental agility. It's simple. Work for 25 minutes and then take a break for 5. Then jump right back in.

But here is a more specific breakdown of the technique itself:

1. Choose a task
2. Set your timer (typically it's 25 minutes, but find your own sweet spot)
3. Work consistently until the timer goes off
4. When the timer goes off, make a checkmark on a piece of paper
5. If you have fewer than 4 checkmarks, take a 5-minute break and repeat step one
6. Once you get to 4 checkmarks, take a break of 15-30 minutes and then start over.

Commitment: Experiment with the Pomodoro technique. If it works for you, keep going. This is a great way to increase productive productivity.

Long-Term Goals

☐
☐
☐
☐
☐
☐
☐
☐
☐

Journal...

Spend On Experiences

"Nothing ever becomes real till it is experienced." — John Keats

To-Do's		Long-Term Goals

We've talked about not prioritizing the acquisition of stuff, and how there are times when frugality can be great, but the truth is that it can be really fun to spend money, and you work hard for your money. So what could you spend it on? Spending on experiences might be the best use of your hard-earned cash.

Taking a trip, seeing a show at the theater, going on a river rafting tour, ziplining, going on a cruise, staying in a log cabin at a ski resort just because it sounds fun—the options are endless. **If you spend your adult life working you'll be able to buy a lot of the stuff you want, but buying things does not create the kinds of memories that experience can.**

And you learn from experiences. And you can share experiences with others.

Commitment: Spend more money on experiences than on things. Make a list of experiences you'd like to experience.

Journal...

Eat At The Table

"Some of the most important conversations I've ever had occurred at my family's dinner table." – Bob Ehrlich

To-Do's
✔
✔
✔
✔
✔
✔
✔
✔

Long-Term Goals

☐
☐
☐
☐
☐
☐
☐
☐

Sitting down and eating at the dinner table, whether done solo or as a family, seems to be a dying art. It's much easier—in more ways than one, sometimes—to eat in front of the TV. It allows you to be passive, multitask, and avoid conversations with other people.

However, you can miss out on some good things if you never sit down together at the table. Meals can have the feeling of a ritual about them. The dinner table is a place to reflect, to grow closer with loved ones, to talk about the day, to laugh, and to eat. And, if you're eating at the table, you probably set the table, and if you set it, there's a good chance that someone prepared food, instead of just grabbing a bag or box of something to eat on the couch.

It's hard for me to imagine anyone regretting more time at the dinner table.

Commitment: Eat at your table more often than you currently do. Preferably with people you love. Make regular family dinners at home a priority.

Journal...

_____
_____
_____
_____
_____
_____
_____
_____
_____
_____
_____
_____
_____
_____
_____
_____
_____
_____
_____
_____
_____
_____

Don't Make People Wait On You

"Better never than late." – George Bernard Shaw

To-Do's		Long-Term Goals

It is really, really obnoxious to wait on people who are habitually late. No matter how well-meaning the person is, or how much we might love him or her, **a person who can't make the effort to be punctual is a person who makes their time more important than the time of the people who are waiting.**

Things happen. Traffic. Flat tires. Trips and falls and illnesses and mild catastrophes with pets and children. Everyone knows this. But that's different from someone who just can't seem to be on time no matter what.

If that's you, there are people who will appreciate your effort to be more punctual. And most of the time, it's not a matter of someone who consciously, callously disregards the time of others. It can just be carelessness or forgetfulness or an inability to concentrate. But we can all do better, and no one can ever resent us for being on time, for any reason.

Commitment: Become more punctual than you are. I like to show up early. This is because there is only one minute during which you are actually on-time. Every minute after that, you're late.

Journal...

October

What Scares You

"I am not afraid of dying. I have lived longer than most people in the world. What scares me is to have a body that works but a brain that is waving goodbye. If that happens, I hope I die quickly." – Henning Mankell

To-Do's
✔
✔
✔
✔
✔
✔
✔
✔

Long-Term Goals

☐ ☐ ☐ ☐ ☐ ☐ ☐ ☐

Fear is generally a signal that says "Stay away!" or "That thing is dangerous!" This makes sense when we're afraid of something plausible like the threat of violence. It makes less sense when we live in the middle of landlocked New Mexico and live in fear of sharks.

Making a list of the things that scare us can be an interesting challenge. **When you see the things you're afraid of, it's hard not to ask why?** If you're afraid of dogs, you might have had a traumatic experience with a dog as a child. But the associations aren't always clear. What if you're afraid of drowning, but you've never even come close?

What if you're afraid of being left by a spouse, or afraid of losing the respect of your child? Where do these fears come from? The better you get at learning the sources of your fear, the better you'll be at overcoming them.

Commitment: Make a fear list. Try to identify when and where each of your fears came from. Once you understand the irrationality of your fears, you will live your life more boldly. Life is too short. Live it boldly.

Journal...

_____
_____
_____
_____
_____
_____
_____
_____
_____
_____
_____
_____
_____
_____
_____
_____
_____
_____
_____
_____

You Can't Always Overcome

"Acceptance of what has happened is the first step to overcoming the consequences of any misfortune." –
William James

To-Do's
✔
✔
✔
✔
✔
✔
✔

Long-Term Goals

☐
☐
☐
☐
☐
☐
☐

Most stories that get billed as inspirational are about people overcoming challenges or setbacks. Hopefully you have some of those stories of your own, because you almost certainly have had challenges and setbacks. But it is also possible to overestimate the importance of overcoming, because it is not always impossible to overcome a challenge.

Sometimes, as in the case of an ongoing illness like Multiple Sclerosis, the best a person can do is to keep going. To try not to let the debilitating disease intrude too much on our daily activities and our lifelong goals. But the disease, or the challenge, or the problems, can always get the upper hand.

All that we can control are our reactions. And our instinctive reactions can always be overcome with diligence.

Commitment: Don't think of overcoming as the goal. Just make sure that you're making progress.

Journal...

Forgive Yourself

"Mistakes are always forgivable, if one has the courage to admit them." – Bruce Lee

To-Do's
✔
✔
✔
✔
✔
✔
✔
✔
✔

You have probably made mistakes. I certainly have. You will probably make more. So will I. And in the aftermath, whether the mistakes are big or small, we will have to decide how we will treat ourselves. Perhaps we'll make justifications for our actions, initially. Maybe we'll beat ourselves up and proclaim ourselves the worst people on earth.

Whatever it looks like in the short term, we must find ways to forgive ourselves. We will live with ourselves, and in our own minds, for, well, as long as we live. **We can't be hospitable to ourselves without forgiveness.** You cannot afford to wield your past mistakes as a club over yourself, or look to them as proof that you're worthless when you're feeling like you have no value.

Forgiveness means to truly let something go. And it can often be harder to forgive ourselves than others. But we have to try.

Commitment: If there is something that you need to forgive yourself for, try to start that process immediately. The simplest thing can be to just write "I forgive you, [insert your name]" over and over again.

Long-Term Goals
☐
☐
☐
☐
☐
☐
☐
☐
☐

Journal...

_____
_____
_____
_____
_____
_____
_____
_____
_____
_____
_____
_____
_____
_____
_____
_____
_____
_____
_____
_____

Take Action

"It is easy to sit up and take notice. What is difficult is getting up and taking action?" – Honore de Balzac

To-Do's		Long-Term Goals
✔		☐
✔		☐
✔		☐
✔		☐
✔		☐
✔		☐
✔		☐
✔		☐

Have you ever heard someone say, "That book changed my life!" Very often, if you pay attention, it is hard to tell if that person's life changed at all. We often talk of being inspired, but we're not actually talking about inspiration unless we truly change the way we think or act as a result of the event. At best, without action, we heard a pep talk.

Nothing happens without action, whether we act or are acted upon. All of the wishing in the world will not bring about the things we want. **Even when the course is unclear, it is generally better to try something than to sit around and hope really hard.**

The discovery of penicillin, the invention of the airplane, the rotary phone, the chair you are currently sitting on, and every other element of progress that the world has experienced, all came about because, at their inception, someone took action.

Commitment: What do you want for yourself? Is there an action you could perform to work towards it? Jot it down in the lines below! Do it now.

Journal...

_____
_____
_____
_____
_____
_____
_____
_____
_____
_____
_____
_____
_____
_____
_____
_____
_____
_____
_____
_____
_____
_____

Improve Your Social Skills

"We're losing social skills, the human interaction skills, how to read a person's mood, to read their body language, how to be patient until the moment is right to make or press a point. Too much exclusive use of electronic information dehumanizes what is a very, very important part of community life and living together."
— Vincent Nichol

To-Do's		Long-Term Goals
✔	The first step to improving your social skills—and we can all improve, whether we're trembling introverts or jetsetters who just want to be the life of the party—is to identify your weaknesses. If you feel awkward in social setting, try to get more specific.	☐
✔		☐
✔	Do you have trouble making eye contact? Coming up with something to say? Do you freeze when someone turns the attention to you? Do your palms sweat at the thought? Do you feel like you say the wrong things? Why? Once you identify your weaknesses you can start working on them. If you have trouble making eye contact, it can be as simple as trying to make more eye contact.	☐
✔		☐
✔		☐
✔	**Other facets of social life can be more challenging and less clear-cut, like dating in the electronic era.** But if you truly want to be better socially, you have to put yourself in social situations and practice. Go easy on yourself, know your limits, but try.	☐
✔		☐
✔	**Commitment:** Identify one social skill that you would like to improve. Put yourself in a social situation this week with the goal of practicing that skill.	☐

Journal...

Get Enough Calories

"Calories from protein affect your brain, your appetite control center, so you are more satiated and satisfied." –
Mark Hyman

To-Do's		Long-Term Goals
✔	One of the benefits of tracking your food intake is that you can monitor if you're getting enough calories for your goals, generally fat loss or muscle gain. But if those aren't goals you're pursuing, there are still reasons to make sure you're getting enough calories.	☐
✔		☐
✔	**Not getting enough calories can make your brain foggy and sap your energy.** It can make it harder just to think and get through the day, forget about trying to get through a workout.	☐
✔		☐
✔	So how much is enough? Well, if you're tracking your calories, you can almost make a note of how you feel that day. Pay attention to how alert you are, or how much energy you have? Do you get sleepier earlier than makes sense to you?	☐
✔		☐
✔	**Commitment:** Get enough calories to suit your goals, whether it's maintaining your weight, gaining, or losing. You really have to track the numbers to make this work. Get an app for your phone that will help you.	☐
✔		☐

Journal...

_____
_____
_____
_____
_____
_____
_____
_____
_____
_____
_____
_____
_____
_____
_____
_____
_____
_____
_____
_____
_____
_____

Get Enough Water

"I never drink water; that is the stuff that rusts pipes." – W.C. Fields

To-Do's

✔

✔

✔

✔

✔

✔

✔

✔

✔

✔

Long-Term Goals

☐

☐

☐

☐

☐

☐

☐

☐

☐

☐

I'm not sure where it started, but you've probably heard that you should drink eight glasses of water a day. It's an arbitrary number that doesn't account for enough variables. But it's true that we each need to try and get enough water each day. I drink around 10 glasses. Water keeps your skin healthy, makes your muscles more full, keep your joints lubricated, and more.

So how much is enough? **An easy rule of thumb is to trust your thirst**, i.e., if you get thirsty, you've gone for too long without water. If you get in the habit of carrying a water bottle with you, or keeping on your desk, it's easy to get more than you're used to by just taking a sip each time you walk by it.

Also, something that usually doesn't get taken into account with the "X amount of ounces per day" crowd is that all liquids are mostly water. Drinking a gallon of diet soda doesn't mean you drank a gallon of healthy water, but it still increases your water intake. But the caffeine will make you urinate most of the water out, so you're actually not helping your water intake.

Commitment: Drink more water than you're used to. Pay attention to how much—and how often—you need to drink in order to never feel thirsty. That's the sweet spot. Also check the color of your urine.

Journal...

_____

_____

_____

_____

_____

_____

_____

_____

_____

_____

_____

_____

_____

_____

_____

_____

_____

_____

Stay Out Of Conversations You're Not Ready For

"People who think they know everything are a great annoyance to those of us who do." – Isaac Asimov

To-Do's		Long-Term Goals

Most know-it-alls are insecure. Something within them says "It's not okay to not know everything. It's not okay to let people think you might not know something." These are the people who cannot stay out of a conversation, no matter what the topic. It's ironic that these people can also be highly intelligent, and may very well know more than others.

But there are few things as useful as *not* being the smartest person in the room. **Or better yet, being in a room where everyone is smarter in some way than we are.** These situations are opportunities for learning that you don't have to create, that don't depend on your willingness to open a book and study. A willingness to defer to the expertise of others is incredibly handy, if you can bear to let other people talk, and you're able to sit back, listen, and learn.

Commitment: If people are talking about things you do not know, there is no reason to be insecure. Just listen and learn. Read up on it later.

Journal...

Let People Like Whatever They Want

"I love criticism just so long as it's unqualified praise." – Noel Coward

To-Do's

✔
✔
✔
✔
✔
✔
✔
✔
✔

Long-Term Goals

☐
☐
☐
☐
☐
☐
☐
☐
☐

Part of becoming an adult is the ability to silence the inner critic. Do you need people to know what you like? If someone mentions a movie or book or song that you don't like, do you really need to tell them that you don't like it? This kind of stuff is for high school, where identities are forming, brains are still developing, and criticism of art rarely goes beyond "I hate it because it's dumb" or "I love it because it's awesome."

There is no accounting for taste. This is why we are lucky enough to have such an eclectic array of humanities. **Culture is not a genre, it is a combination of the ideas and art of anyone in the society.** How boring would it be if the style of music that I loved was the only one there was? Or literature? Or film?

You would probably never do anything on purpose to hurt someone's feelings. But this is what happens on some level when we criticize something just because we don't like it. Well, someone else *does* like it, and each of our reactions can be right, even if we don't talk about it.

Commitment: Avoid criticizing what other people like. You can have a critic's temperament without needing to weigh in on everything.

Journal...

Know The Forms Of Poverty

"Loneliness and the feeling of being unwanted is the most terrible poverty." – Mother Theresa

To-Do's		Long-Term Goals

There is more to poverty than simply not having enough money. And even then, living in true financial poverty is different than not having enough money. **But there are more forms of poverty than the one with dollar signs attached to it, and they can be even more devastating to a happy life.**

Someone who lives in emotional poverty may experience crushing loneliness. This might be a person without a friend, or without family. Or someone who is unable to bond emotionally with people, or feels misunderstood. Someone who is mocked or bullied. Intellectual poverty is real as well. A person whose mind is never stimulated, whether through their own choices, or by uncontrollable circumstances, is also living below a different type of poverty line.

As with so many of the tips in this book, understanding the types of poverty you may be dealing with will require self-scrutiny and diligence. And as with so many of the tips in this book, it will require you to think deeply.

Commitment: Identify the forms of poverty in your life. Write them down. Take whatever steps you can to correct them. Ask someone, who has what you're wanting, for help.

Journal...

Be Frugal

"Polaroid by its nature makes you frugal. You walk around with maybe two packs of film in your pocket. You have 20 shots, so each shot is a world." – Patti Smith

To-Do's		Long-Term Goals
✔		☐
✔		☐
✔		☐
✔		☐
✔		☐
✔		☐
✔		☐
✔		☐

We all work hard, and deserve to hang onto the money we earn. But even if we are careful and don't overspend extravagantly, it is nearly always possible to be more frugal than we are. This is not to suggest an Ebenezer Scrooge level of miserliness, but rather, a heightened sense of attention to our spending habits.

Do you finish all of the food you buy? Do you buy new books or clothes when you could buy used? Do you replace your phone before it's necessary because you want to have the latest model, even though the latest model might not be any more useful than the previous one? Do you waste toothpaste or shampoo or shaving cream? Could you work out at home instead of paying for a gym membership? I call these small money drips...stopping them won't make you rich, but you won't be surprised by the bill at the end of the month.

The point is that there are always more questions to ask ourselves. Frugality will never feel like a mistake.

Commitment: Find ways to cut out small money drips.

Journal...

October 12

Don't Take The Criticism (Or The Praise) Literally

"The trouble with most of us is that we would rather be ruined by praise than saved by criticism." — Norman Vincent Peale

To-Do's
✔
✔
✔
✔
✔
✔
✔
✔
✔

Long-Term Goals

☐ ☐ ☐ ☐ ☐ ☐ ☐ ☐ ☐

One of the best lessons a writer can learn is that you shouldn't take the praise, or the criticism, personally. Now, this refers to the criticism of a piece of writing. If someone tells you your writing is wonderful, you want to believe them. You might start to think you are every bit as good as people tell you you are, and maybe you really are!

On the other hand, when people criticize a piece of writing, or tell you that it's horrible, it's more natural for an author to get defensive, or to think that the person just didn't "get it." But if you hear that you're a bad writer often enough, you might start to believe that as well.

The truth is, you only have the words you send out into the world. You forfeit other peoples' reactions to them. If the writing is good, it's not because other people say it's good. If it's bad, it's not because of other people saying it's bad. You can extend this parallel to all forms of praise and criticism. **You are you because you're *you*, not because of what anyone says you are.**

Commitment: Enjoy the praise, embrace the criticism, don't take either personally. Keep being true to your highest self.

Journal...

Get A Baloney Detection Kit

"Skepticism: the mark and even the pose of the educated mind." – John Dewey

To-Do's		Long-Term Goals

Skepticism can be useful to anyone, even the most devout person of faith. **A mind that cannot question has, in some ways, ceased to be a mind.** Skepticism is not a dogma, but a simple method with which to ask questions when a claim is presented. It is a very useful way to look at a statement and figure out how to approach it, and whether you can believe it or not.

I've never seen the benefits of skepticism laid out more gently—because there are plenty of skeptics who can only operate in sneering, condescending, attack mode—than Carl Sagan did in his playful articles on what he called "Baloney Detection."

It is a mind-expanding way to probe at questions and to try to outsmart your own arguments. Rather than belabor it here, I'll move on to the commitment and let Sagan speak for himself.

Commitment: Read Carl Sagan's *The Fine Art of Baloney Detection.* It's short and easy to find online.

Journal...

Don't Focus On The 1%

"It is not strange... to mistake change for progress." – Millard Fillmore

To-Do's

- ✔
- ✔
- ✔
- ✔
- ✔
- ✔
- ✔
- ✔
- ✔
- ✔

Long-Term Goals

- ☐
- ☐
- ☐
- ☐
- ☐
- ☐
- ☐
- ☐
- ☐

When people are trying to gain muscle, 99% of their progress comes from three things: lifting heavy (for them) weights, eating enough food, and getting enough sleep. If these three things are happening, progress is inevitable. However, it's tempting to believe that there are quick fixes and shortcuts, and **quick fixes and shortcuts are the dreams of the 1%.**

The 1% says that what you need is a fancier program, not the basics of lifting, eating, and sleeping. The 1% says that there is a supplement that will jumpstart you and make you look like someone on a magazine cover in four weeks. The 1% says that it's not that your fundamentals are out of whack, it's that you're doing the wrong rep scheme or not getting stability work or not balancing often enough on a Bosu ball.

This isn't just about getting stronger. Any facet of life has its equivalent of the 1% and the 99%. Until you are doing the 99%, there is no reason to get hung up on the 1%.

Commitment: Do the 99% first, and do it for as long as it takes. These are the fundamentals. Then, when you finally plateau, get into the 1%.

Journal...

Define Fitness

"Fitness needs to be perceived as fun and games or we subconsciously avoid it." – Alan Thicke

To-Do's		Long-Term Goals
✔	The more specific a goal is, the simpler it is to pursue. Not easy, but simple, as in, specificity takes out a lot of the guesswork. Unfortunately, many people don't make specific goals. For instance, "I want to get in shape," or "I want to be fit," sound specific, but they're not. Let's define what fitness actually is.	☐
✔		☐
✔	Being "fit" is not a thing. **Being fit to do *a specific task* is.** A forklift driver is fit to drive a forklift. A powerlifter is fit to perform the three big lifts at a powerlifting meet. A ballerina is fit to dance ballet. When most people talk about fitness, they're talking about looking good, having a certain standard of cardiovascular health, losing weight, or being more muscular. But these are better examples of being healthier, not necessarily of having achieved a vague idea of "fitness."	☐
✔		☐
✔		☐
✔		☐
✔	**Commitment:** Make your goals as specific as possible. Decide what fitness means to you, and think about it in specific terms.	☐

Journal...

Make A Time Capsule (Or At Least Think About It)

"We seem to have a compulsion these days to bury time capsules in order to give those people living in the next century or so some idea of what we are like." – Alfred Hitchcock

To-Do's		Long-Term Goals

Back in elementary school, did you ever make a time capsule? The idea is that you would fill a capsule—think of a cylinder about the size of a fire hydrant—with things from that year. Whoever unearthed it in the future would be able to open it and say "Ah! So that's what things were like back then!"

If you were going to fill a time capsule with things about *you,* with the understanding that you must try to distill yourself for whoever finds it 50 years later, what would you put inside of it? **What would you want people to know about you?**

This exercise can be great at showing when we're just going through the motions. If your day is basically going to work and then Netflix at night, this thought experiment might give you something to think about.

Commitment: Imagine making a time capsule. Choose 12 things that you would put inside of it that would show someone in the future who you were.

Journal...

Read Certain Books

"A book is a dream that you hold in your hand." – Neil Gaiman

To-Do's		Long-Term Goals

This is not going to be a list of the books that you should reread. Rather, this is a prompt to think about the books that have meant the most to you. Books that you remember fondly, or books that are simply unforgettable to you. Books that changed the way you thought or acted.

Now, once you have a few of them, reread them. Really pay attention to whether they seem to have changed. Obviously, they haven't, the words are always the words, but perhaps *you* have changed. **The lens through which you view life is altered by experiences and days lived.**

You might feel different things, or notice different things. If nothing else, if you reread a book every five years, your memory will be five years older and much of the book will seem fresh to you again.

Commitment: Choose three books that have been meaningful to you and read them again. For me, I reread *Think and Grow Rich* by Napolean Hill; *Love in the Time of Cholera* by Marquez; and *Too Soon Old, Too Late Smart* by Gordon Livingston.

Journal...

Listen To New (For You) Types Of Music

"Music is part of being human." – Oliver Sacks

To-Do's		Long-Term Goals

Music is an odd thing. Darwin was mystified by it, as he could find no explanation for the human propensity to enjoy listening to, and creating, what are essentially meaningless patterns of tones and rhythms. But music is a multi-billion-dollar industry. We listen to it for pleasure, for inspiration, for diversion during our commutes. **And I suspect that most people are genuinely affected by music, even if they can't explain its effect on them.**

I would suggest that we should listen to whatever has the power to move us. For that reason, it can be worth trying to branch out into different forms of music, even though we all have our favorite styles. Take a week and experiment with different genres—and these days there is a dizzying array of subgenres. Techno, country, electronica, R&B, rock in all its forms, music across all the centuries. And there's so much more.

Expand your musical horizons. You might find something that really moves you in mysterious ways...(a shout-out to U2.)

Commitment: Musically, take a week to listen to a style that you're unfamiliar with.

Journal...

Keep Track Of The Books You Read

"Reading is a basic tool in the living of a good life." – Joseph Addison

To-Do's

- ✔
- ✔
- ✔
- ✔
- ✔
- ✔
- ✔
- ✔

Long-Term Goals

- ☐
- ☐
- ☐
- ☐
- ☐
- ☐
- ☐
- ☐

There was a very sad poll—too depressing to link to, but trust me—a couple of years ago that said if you had read six books that year, you could call yourself "well-read." Six! Six is certainly better than zero, but it's a pretty low bar. This is because the average American reads only 1 book a year. Anyhow, one of the best ways to make sure you're reading more than six books is to keep track of the books you read.

If you can look back at what you were reading ten years ago, it might say more about you than any journal could. Reading habits change, tastes change, we discover new subjects and others. Sometimes the reading list reflects a soul that was dark and moody, or one that was binging on self-help books. There are phases of light and phases of silliness. Fiction and nonfiction. It can really be fascinating if you give yourself a chance to look back at your reading habits. Highly recommended.

Commitment: Start a reading notebook, or join a literary social network like Goodreads.

Journal...

October 20

Don't Push Through Pain

"The aim of the wise is not to secure pleasure, but to avoid pain." – Aristotle

To-Do's		Long-Term Goals

Of all the backwards training philosophies, "No pain, no gain," might be the worst. The Internet has worked wonders for the sharing of information, but it has also made it easier to share the worst sort of misinformation. Do a quick Google search for inspirational fitness or weightlifting quotes and you'll run into inanities like, "Crawling is acceptable. Puking is acceptable. Tears are acceptable. Pain is acceptable. Quitting is unacceptable."

This is idiocy. **We all have limitations.** We all have different ages and injury histories. There is a massive difference between exerting extreme amounts of effort during a strength training session or a grueling run, and continuing to work while you're in damage mode. Exercise can be hard and that's fine.

But *it shouldn't hurt* and *it shouldn't leave you in pain.* Know your limits, respect the signals your body gives you, and ignore anyone who tells you that you're weak for respecting your body.

Commitment: Forget about "No pain, no gain" and focus on achieving *consistent* results.

Journal...

Go For A Climb

"It is not the mountain we conquer but ourselves." – Edmund Hillary

To-Do's		Long-Term Goals

✔

✔

✔

✔

✔

✔

✔

✔

✔

Going for a hike, or honestly, doing any sort of climb, can feel like play. Hiking up a mountain, or scaling one, if you're more adventurous, is exercise that stops feeling like exercise. It gives you a chance to get out in nature, and to take your body to places it probably doesn't go very often.

But let's say you don't have any mountains. Even if you live in the flattest stretch of Kansas, you might be able to find a climbing gym. Learning to move across the face of a rock wall in a supervised climbing gym where you're totally safe and someone can train you, is exhilarating in a way that can't be explained, it simply must be experienced.

Climbing can also be scaled to the abilities of the individual, but everything about it is useful. The pulling, pushing, endurance, and body control required are unlike any other activity. But trust me, once you hit the peak of a famous top, like Kilimanjaro, you will be awed. Not only will your body be challenged but also your understanding of what is "magnificent" will be severely shaken.

Commitment: Start working climbing of some sort into your fitness routine. Consider an adventure using one of Dean Cardinale's climbing excursions at wwtrek.com. You won't regret it.

☐ ☐ ☐ ☐ ☐ ☐ ☐ ☐ ☐

Journal...

You Can Always Close The Laptop

"People take things at face value on social media. Earnestness is the assumption." – Mindy Kaling

To-Do's
✔
✔
✔
✔
✔
✔
✔
✔

Long-Term Goals

☐ ☐ ☐ ☐ ☐ ☐ ☐ ☐

Arguing with someone can be exhausting, frustrating, even frightening at times, depending on your tolerance for confrontation. But when a conversation ends, at least you can get away from the person and start to recover. It's not always so easy when the confrontation, or argument, or bullying is taking place online.

You *know* that the comment, or Facebook post, or email is sitting there, waiting for you to look at it again, to stew about it, to respond and *prove* to the other person that you're right. There are more ways than ever to keep a conversation going, which can be great unless it's a conversation that you're trying to end.

Just keep in mind that you can always close the laptop. You can always turn off your phone. **It is the same as walking away from a person you don't want to argue with.**

Commitment: The next time you're tempted to respond to something negative online, just don't. Fight the agitation it causes you. The more often you resist, the easier it will get.

Journal...

Learn Basic Internet Fluency

"We are all now connected by the Internet, like neurons in a giant brain." – Stephen Hawking

To-Do's

- ✔
- ✔
- ✔
- ✔
- ✔
- ✔
- ✔
- ✔
- ✔

Long-Term Goals

- ☐
- ☐
- ☐
- ☐
- ☐
- ☐
- ☐
- ☐
- ☐

Every tax season, a new group of disgruntled people arise: people who don't want to do their taxes online, or who just want the tax forms and booklets like before. Similar laments take place in libraries every day, where people shake their heads sadly and say "Well, it's all going online."

In many ways, it's true, and this pattern is not going to reverse itself. **So, no matter how much we might groan and long for the way things were, we aren't going back to the days of dial-up.** And because the online world is so entrenched now—it's really hard to even find a phone option that *isn't* a smartphone, try it—it's a good idea to learn the basics. Understand how email works. Learn how a web browser and search engine work.

Most people will honestly never *need* the vast majority of what the Internet and computers are capable of. But you'll have fewer headaches if you know how to do a few simple things. Think about this—computers are going away. Eventually every surface we touch will be a searchable surface that connects us to the internet.

Commitment: Learn basic internet skills. Most local libraries offer computer classes. Or ask a friend or family member for a crash course.

Journal...

Autopay Your Bills

"It is essential that we stop worrying about money and stop resenting our bills." – Louise L. Hay

To-Do's		Long-Term Goals

Life can turn into a storm of bills. There are so many things to keep track of and to pay for. And unpaid bills, whether they go unpaid through carelessness or financial hardships, result in bigger bills and damaged credit. This is a process worth simplifying and making foolproof for the forgetful. **Think of your bills as a form of trust—someone believed in you enough that they were willing to provide a service first without being paid.** In this way, bills are blessings, not curses.

It's rare these days to find a bill that does not have an autopay option. Insurance, credit cards, auto loans, Netflix, Internet, telephone, etc. As long as you can make sure that you have money in your account when the bills get processed through autopay, you don't have to do anything else. It saves a world of potential headaches and your bills never snowball, because they never go unpaid for even a month.

Commitment: Set as many of your bills as possible to autopay.

Journal...

Donate Blood If You Can

"The best blood will at some time get into a fool or a mosquito." – Austin O'Malley

To-Do's
✔
✔
✔
✔
✔
✔
✔
✔

Hopefully you never need a blood transfusion. But if you do, the blood will be available because someone donated it. Blood is not grown in a lab, or purchased in a store. It is donated by people who care enough to want to help others down the road.

Donating blood is an easy way to make a difference. And if you have a rare blood type, it is all the more important that you donate blood if you can. There are regular blood drives in most areas, and it is always possible to find somewhere to donate when there's not an ongoing blood drive.

It is a way to literally save someone's life. **And someone out there is donating today in the hopes that their generous act will help someone like you or me, should we ever need it.**

Commitment: Donate blood the next time you have a chance. Scientists are feverishly working on blood substitutes, but at the publication of this book, we currently do have any other viable options.

Long-Term Goals
☐
☐
☐
☐
☐
☐
☐
☐

Journal...

Try You Prove Yourself Wrong

"Differences challenge assumptions." – Anne Wilson Schaef

To-Do's

- ✓
- ✓
- ✓
- ✓
- ✓
- ✓
- ✓
- ✓
- ✓
- ✓
- ✓

Long-Term Goals

- ☐
- ☐
- ☐
- ☐
- ☐
- ☐
- ☐
- ☐
- ☐
- ☐
- ☐

It is very easy to spot when others are wrong. In fact, I wouldn't be surprised if lots of people have more conviction about why other people are wrong, than in why they themselves are right. And if you have strongly held beliefs—and hopefully you do—it can be hard, or seem downright counterproductive, to question them periodically.

But true reasoning is the act of trying to take apart your own arguments, not those of others. It is to look closely at your own data and arguments and beliefs, and to try to identify your blind spots, or to see where your own logic breaks down. The uncomfortable part of this is that, if you see that you've been wrong about something, now you must make a choice: **change your behavior or thinking accordingly, or keep going with a train of thought that you now know to be questionable, if not outright wrong.**

If you can stomach it, make a list of things you believe to be true. They don't have to be spiritual; it can just be anything you believe to be true that is important to you. If they are based on tradition—something like, "I believe this because my mother told me"—try figuring out if there are more reasons for believing. Try to figure out how/if you might be wrong.

Commitment: Simply commit to making the list, examining your truths, and being as honest and open about the task as possible. You will learn something.

Journal...

You Can't Plan For Anything

"Planning is bringing the future into the present so that you can do something about it now." – Alan Lakein

To-Do's

- ✔
- ✔
- ✔
- ✔
- ✔
- ✔
- ✔
- ✔
- ✔
- ✔

Long-Term Goals

- ☐
- ☐
- ☐
- ☐
- ☐
- ☐
- ☐
- ☐
- ☐

It's good to have a plan for your life. Financial, emotional, physical, spiritual—the more detailed the plan, the better your results will be, if you have the discipline to follow the plan. And yet, plans go awry. Circumstances and catastrophes and the hassles of normal life intrude and combine to smash our plans to smithereens.

Which is why **it's also valuable to acknowledge that your plan is going to change.** If you're working on your adaptability, you'll be able to roll with the punches, or at least to do so as well as anyone can when things get hard. Recognizing that the plan will change is never a reason to minimize the value of planning, or to abandon the idea altogether.

You will proceed with your life as best you can, based on the information you have and the circumstances you're presented with. Some will be controllable. Some will not. Whatever happens, having a plan will help you make as much progress as possible, until things change.

Commitment: Make a detailed plan for your life, revisit it frequently, and prepare yourself for the day it changes.

Journal...

Move Your Alarm Clock

"I like things that are simple, such as an alarm clock." – Morgan Freeman

To-Do's
✔
✔
✔
✔
✔
✔
✔

Ideally, you don't have to wake up to an alarm clock. If you get summoned from sleep by anything that dings or beeps or buzzes or vibrates, you could probably use more sleep. Alas, most of us adhere to schedules that are not always kind to our rest.

When an alarm clock—or your phone, whatever you use—is within arm's reach, it can be all too easy to turn it off without getting out of bed. Then, maybe you fall back asleep. Or maybe you spend time zoning out on your smartphone when you could be up doing something useful, like eating breakfast or sparing yourself more of a rush than is necessary.

If you put your alarm clock across the room, you'll have to get up to turn it off. Simple and effective.

Commitment: Put your alarm clock across the room. Read *The Miracle Morning* by Hal Elrod, and get more out of your early morning ritual.

Long-Term Goals
☐
☐
☐
☐
☐
☐
☐

Journal...

There Are Lots Of Ways To Vent

"I pray on the principle that wine knocks the cork out of a bottle. There is an inward fermentation, and there must be a vent." – Henry Ward Beecher

To-Do's		Long-Term Goals

✔

✔

✔

✔

✔

✔

✔

✔

✔

✔

"Thanks, I just needed to vent." If you've ever heard that, you probably just got done listening to someone go off on a tirade. Maybe it was about their boss, or a spouse, or a political party, or money trouble. The point is, venting usually takes a verbal form, and sometimes we all need it. Venting is different than whining. Venting is about letting off steam in a sustained burst, rather than bottling it up until it explodes.

However, venting doesn't always make you feel better. **It can be draining and doesn't always lead to a solution.** Venting is usually just a chance to say something that you can't afford to say in public, or to the people who might most need to hear it. But there are also other ways to vent.

When you've got that frantic frustration, there are always ways to diffuse the energy. Run. Do pushups. Go for a walk. Do hill sprints. Pull weeds like a maniac. Do yoga. Remember, venting is about the release of pressure. Any form of distraction might serve just as well as spilling your guts to someone, although I don't want you to discount the value of that as well.

Commitment: There's no perfect way to vent, but keep in mind that there are options besides a stream of consciousness rant. Verbal rants can lead to unintended consequences. Keep experimenting with non-vocal alternatives.

☐ ☐ ☐ ☐ ☐ ☐ ☐ ☐ ☐ ☐

Journal...

Be Realistic About Your Disciplines

"A lack of realism in the vision today costs credibility tomorrow." – John C. Maxwell

To-Do's		Long-Term Goals

To-Do's
- ✔
- ✔
- ✔
- ✔
- ✔
- ✔
- ✔
- ✔
- ✔

Long-Term Goals
- ☐
- ☐
- ☐
- ☐
- ☐
- ☐
- ☐
- ☐
- ☐

I once heard a powerlifter joke that he was going to write a book called *48 Months To The Body Of Your Dreams.* The joke is that it's a pretty realistic title, and that no one would want to buy it. 48 months? The magazines all say that I'm only three weeks from putting three inches on my arms, losing 20 pounds of fat, while gaining 30 pounds of muscle!

If you want a body that looks like it took 10 years to build, it may take 10 years of disciplined training to build it. If you want to put 100 pounds on your bench press, it might take two years, not three weeks. If you want to lose 100 pounds, it isn't going to come off overnight, no matter what the latest celebrity trainer on *The Biggest Loser* says.

Yes, genetics matter. Yes, age matters. **But the only thing we can always control is the discipline we're willing to apply to make the best progress that each of us can make.** So shoot big, make goals, and be unrealistic in those goals, but be *realistic* in your discipline. It will take "every day" discipline. Many, many small steps will eventually lead to massive progress.

Commitment: Be bold in your goals and grand vision. Also, be realistic about your level of discipline. We all have limits, and it will take much more discipline than you believe.

Journal...

Do Something Spooky

"I love Halloween, and I love that feeling: the cold air, the spooky dangers lurking around the corner." – Evan Peters

To-Do's

- ✔
- ✔
- ✔
- ✔
- ✔
- ✔
- ✔
- ✔
- ✔

Long-Term Goals

- ☐
- ☐
- ☐
- ☐
- ☐
- ☐
- ☐
- ☐
- ☐

Today is a day to celebrate things that go bump in the night. In his book *On Writing,* horror master Stephen King said that he wasn't sure exactly why he gravitated to dark material, but he always had "a love of the unquiet coffin." Now, you don't have to read horror novels, put on a mask, go trick or treating, or howl at the moon tonight. But, I would encourage you to take part in the fun and do something spooky.

Unless the idea is totally repulsive to you, take a local ghost tour. Visit a haunted house, whether it's a house that is rumored to be haunted, or one of the scare fests where you buy a ticket and things jump out at you as you go through the rooms. Watch a scary movie. Read a ghost story. Get some friends together and *tell* ghost stories.

But **take part in the fun.** It's what just about everyone else will be doing tonight. Halloween is an easy way to reintroduce a childlike sense of play back into your life, if only for a night.

Commitment: Do something worthy of Halloween tonight. Dress up. Decorate your house. Go to a costume party. Make a spooky memory with someone you love.

Journal...

November

Know What Supplements Are, And What They Aren't

"I need protein from food rather than just protein supplements." – Travis Barker

To-Do's		Long-Term Goals

To-Do's
- ✔
- ✔
- ✔
- ✔
- ✔
- ✔

If you walk into a GNC you will see an array of the shriekiest ad copy imaginable. Everything is "hardcore." Everything is "essential." And yet, the question few people seem to ask is, "Essential to what?" GNC sells supplements. And here's another question: "What are they supplements for?"

Supplements add to or enhance something that is already there. **By definition, supplements are not a foundation.** But in the shortcut-obsessed world of fitness and fat loss, supplements are the one thing you "must" have. They're supplements! They are the cherry on top that might get you a little edge in peak performance, *if* you're already sleeping enough, eating enough good food, and exercising enough.

Commitment: Before you put supplements on a pedestal, make sure everything else in your routine—nutrition and exercise—is squared away.

Long-Term Goals
- ☐
- ☐
- ☐
- ☐
- ☐
- ☐

Journal...

November 2

What Is The Meaning Of Life?

"You will never be happy if you continue to search for what happiness consists of. You will never live if you are looking for the meaning of life." – Albert Camus

To-Do's
✔
✔
✔
✔
✔
✔
✔
✔
✔

In Douglas Adams's novel *The Hitchhiker's Guide To The Galaxy,* the question "What is the answer to the ultimate question of life, the universe, and everything?" Is asked of a supercomputer called Deep Thought. It takes over seven million years to compute the answer, which is given on a feverishly anticipated day. But the answer is "42." This is a disappointment to the truth seekers, but the computer maintains that they asked the wrong question.

And yet, we continue to ask what the meaning of life is. Many religions and philosophies answer the question with specific frameworks and ideologies and creation stories, but there is rampant disagreement among them all. **The question is perhaps best posed by each of us, to ourselves.**

Ultimately, it is up to us to decide what is meaningful, and then to fill our lives with meaningful things and meaningful adventures. This is comforting and liberating to some, and frightening to others. As with many things in this book, it is all a matter of perspective.

Commitment: Know what the meaning of *your* life is. Think, think, and act accordingly.

Long-Term Goals

☐ ☐ ☐ ☐ ☐ ☐ ☐ ☐

Journal...

Rehab Your Injuries

"The more injuries you get, the smarter you get." – Mikhail Baryshnikov

To-Do's

✔

✔

✔

✔

✔

✔

✔

✔

Long-Term Goals

☐
☐
☐
☐
☐
☐
☐
☐

We all pick up lingering pains and aches as we age. Things we have to work around, at least temporarily. But, while we tend to bounce back slower from injuries—minor or major—as we age, we can't just ignore these pains and push through them just because it would be inconvenient to do otherwise. Pushing through pain and exacerbating injuries is more inconvenient in the long term.

When you have an injury, you need to rehab it as much as possible before resuming the sort of movements and activities that caused the injury. This could mean simply taking a rest, icing it, using anti-inflammatories, seeing a chiropractor, or doing physical therapy. **But most of the time, thinking you can just work through it is a recipe for more pain**. And pain tends to lead to pain, as the body overcompensates for structures that are weakened or out of alignment.

Commitment: The next time you have a lingering pain, *do not make it worse*. Figure out how to rehab it. Your body will thank you.

Journal...

Anything Is Possible If You Do It Slowly

"And that's been my motto in life. You can do anything. You just do it slowly enough." – Lauren Groff

✔

✔

✔

✔

✔

✔

✔

☐
☐
☐
☐
☐
☐
☐

Lauren Gross is the author of several big, audacious, intricately plotted books that many authors would give an arm to have written. But her method is simple—she is thoughtful, and she does not go faster than would be beneficial to the work. There are obviously exceptions to the rule—Olympic lifters, for example, require speed above all else to perform their sport.

But generally speaking, anything that takes care and diligence, no matter how daunting the task may seem, can be accomplished if you do it slowly. How slowly? Results will vary. **But slowly *enough.*** You know when you're rushing through something. So do I. And we both probably know when it affects our work or our thoughts. Couple pace with persistence and you have a formula for success.

Commitment: Slow down. Remember Groff's quote. If you want an example of her motto in action, read her novel *Fates And Furies.*

Journal...

Always Start Out Positive When Someone Comes Home

"It takes one person to forgive, it takes two people to be reunited." – Lewis B. Smedes

To-Do's

- ✔
- ✔
- ✔
- ✔
- ✔
- ✔
- ✔
- ✔

Long-Term Goals

- ☐
- ☐
- ☐
- ☐
- ☐
- ☐
- ☐
- ☐

Have you ever come home—or met someone somewhere else—and had them lay into you with the latest saga, in a wash of negativity? It can really deflate the mood, particularly if you're coming home to a significant other. It completely takes the focus off of you, and makes you an immediate audience without asking if you needed time to decompress.

You may have done this to someone else as well. If so, you know how it feels, and you certainly wouldn't want to do it to someone more often than necessary. Even where there are hard matters to discuss, or you need to vent, there is nearly always a way to start out positive. Smile, embrace, do a brief recap of the day, and then ask if you can have a serious talk. At that point, any of the negativity that may necessarily accompany the conversation will be softened, and you'll have a more attentive listener.

Commitment: Don't start out any interaction by unloading all of the problems immediately. Welcome them home first. Start positive, then say what you have to say.

Journal...

Take Your Country's Citizenship Exam

"Citizenship is a tough occupation which obliges the citizen to make his own informed opinion and stand by it."
– Martha Gellhorn

To-Do's
✔
✔
✔
✔
✔
✔
✔
✔

Long-Term Goals

☐
☐
☐
☐
☐
☐
☐
☐

If you've never looked at your country's citizenship exam, you might overestimate how much you know about the basics of your civics structure. Google "Sample questions for citizenship exam" and see how many you can answer. Much like babies stop crawling when they learn how to walk, it can be easy to let the foundational knowledge of a state slide when we're no longer being asked to name capitals or give social studies reports on the House versus The Senate.

When my father and I went for our citizenships, he studied and fretted over the exam, while I took the knowledge for granted. I'm happy to say that we both passed the exam, but I was quite surprised by how difficult the study questions were.

I think you too will be surprised.

Commitment: Try the citizenship exam. If you're behind the curve, do what you need to do in order to know enough to get a passing grade. Take pride in your country's history.

Journal...

Make Something

"Creativity takes courage." – Henri Matisse

To-Do's

- ✔
- ✔
- ✔
- ✔
- ✔
- ✔
- ✔
- ✔

Long-Term Goals

- ☐
- ☐
- ☐
- ☐
- ☐
- ☐
- ☐
- ☐

Most kids I have known are instinctively creative. They are *driven* to make things, whether it's drawing pictures, painting, making sand castles, or even making messes as they destroy yet another tower of blocks. They seem to get a huge kick out of seeing something and knowing: *I made that.*

This instinct is in everyone, but circumstances conspire to take away our time. Sometimes the creative instinct gets stifled. Stifled long enough and then...maybe it goes away. **But it can always be retrieved.** This is the simple truth, even if you've forgotten—it is fun to make things.

It is fun to point at something and say "That was not here before I was." This is why I've always appreciated great art, architecture, music, or design.

Commitment: Make something. Some piece of art, whether it's visual, a piece of writing, or a sand castle. Do it as best as you can and don't take yourself too seriously. Gather a group and do a "wine and paint" class.

Journal...

Remember What You Want

"You can do what you want to do. You can be what you want to be." – Dave Thomas

To-Do's

- ✔
- ✔
- ✔
- ✔
- ✔
- ✔
- ✔
- ✔

Long-Term Goals

- ☐
- ☐
- ☐
- ☐
- ☐
- ☐
- ☐
- ☐

With all of the business in your life, do you take enough time to do what you want? It's sort of a trick question, because in order to want something, you have to know what you want. Which requires contemplation and planning, two things that don't always fit into a hectic life.

But if we owe ourselves anything, it is a shot at getting what we want. Ironically, it is often by doing what we don't want that we learn what we *do* want, as long as we take time to sit still for a second and remind ourselves of the things we want.

A week becomes a month quickly. The years fly by. If you are going to go through the rough and tumble business of living, you deserve to chase the things you want while you're at it.

Commitment: Remember what you want. Don't let yourself forget. Write it down in your journal every day. Consider posting reminders in places where you will see them frequently. I keep a list of my wants in my wallet.

Journal...

Better Than Getting Defensive

"My defensiveness in life really helps me as a driver." – Larry David

To-Do's
✔
✔
✔
✔
✔
✔
✔
✔
✔

Long-Term Goals

☐ ☐ ☐ ☐ ☐ ☐ ☐ ☐ ☐

If you feel defensive when you're accused of something, or when someone says something about you that's not true, you're not alone. It is natural to want to defend ourselves. But it's not always in our best interests. Now, there is a different side to this which is the point of this tip.

If you feel defensive because two, or three, or five, or fifty people, or *everyone* seems to be saying the same thing about you, there might be a better route. Namely, "I wonder why they might think that?" **There is a point at which we need to ask ourselves whether something about our perceptions might be off.** When the same feedback comes in over and over, it's time for an honest look at ourselves.

This doesn't necessarily feel better than getting defensive, but it's going to be more useful in the long run.

Commitment: When you find yourself getting defensive about the same thing, over and over, ask yourself instead what might be prompting people to say it. Understand that all problems arise from within. Start there. Always look within first.

Journal...

Make Room In Your Closet

"There's a lot of skeletons in my closet, but I know what they're wearing. I'm not gonna act all ashamed of it." – Naomi Watts

To-Do's

- ✔
- ✔
- ✔
- ✔
- ✔
- ✔
- ✔
- ✔
- ✔
- ✔

Long-Term Goals

- ☐
- ☐
- ☐
- ☐
- ☐
- ☐
- ☐
- ☐
- ☐
- ☐

It happens slowly. A closet that gets tighter, and tighter, and soon you're wedging hangers and clothes in. The same can happen to a dresser drawer. And then you're dealing with a sort of clutter that can be hard for some people to let go of. People who would never leave a floor unswept or a flat surface covered in knick knacks will still quibble at the thought of getting rid of some old, unworn clothes.

Here is an easy guideline: if you haven't worn it in three months, consider letting it go. Donate it to a used clothing store, sell it if you wear the kind of clothes that people would buy, or *start wearing it again.* The obvious exception is if you have a lot of seasonal clothes and you're just not going to wear them every three months.

A clean closet can free up a lot of headspace. Old clothes carry with them old memories, which are not always positive memories. Yes, old clothes can be a form of negative energy. So free yourself by getting rid of them. And if nothing else, it makes room for more new clothes.

Commitment: Give your closet a cleaning. If three months seems too arbitrary an amount, pick something that makes more sense to you. Donate them to your favorite organization. Don't even bother with a garage sale, for old clothes don't typically sell well.

Journal...

_____
_____
_____
_____
_____
_____
_____
_____
_____
_____
_____
_____
_____
_____
_____
_____
_____
_____
_____

Walk With Confidence

"Life is not easy for any of us. But what of that? We must have perseverance and above all confidence in ourselves. We must believe that we are gifted for something and that this thing must be attained." – Marie Curie

To-Do's
✔
✔
✔
✔
✔
✔
✔
✔

When you think of someone confident, what do you picture? Is it their tone of voice? Are they smiling? Do they make eye contact? Are they socially gregarious? And, how do they walk? **You might be picturing someone with a long stride, who seems to know exactly where they're going.**

Body language isn't everything, but it isn't *nothing* either. The way we walk is a signal. You will never see someone slouching, stooped, dragging their feet with their eyes on the ground, and think "Wow! What a confident person!" But if someone is walking confidently, you can see it from a block away.

Be that person. At the very least, walking confidently requires good posture. Chin up, shoulders back, arms swinging naturally, and shoulders down. And the more you walk confidently, the more confident you will feel.

Commitment: Walk with confidence. Remind yourself consistently and it will soon be a habit that you don't have to think about.

Long-Term Goals
☐
☐
☐
☐
☐
☐
☐
☐

Journal...

November 12

You Can't Spot Reduce

"There's a huge emotional component to weight loss." – Carnie Wilson

To-Do's

- ✔
- ✔
- ✔
- ✔
- ✔
- ✔
- ✔
- ✔
- ✔

"Spot reduction" refers to the idea of losing fat in a specific area, as a result of a specific exercise. For instance, if marketing ads have taught us anything, it's that the secret to having a flat stomach is doing crunches. Except, it's not. No amount of crunches will take the fat off of our stomachs. Crunches simply build the muscle beneath the fat. If the fat stays, you'll never see the new muscle.

Fat loss is not specific to any areas of the body. There are some exceptions—some people are more likely to carry extra weight in their stomach, or thighs, or upper arms—but if you actually want to get lean, provisionally accept that you need to lose weight all over, because *that's the only way it happens.* **Weight gain and weight loss are distributed all over.**

The only way to get slimmer arms, or a leaner torso, or more slender thighs, or to zap those love handles, is to lose weight. Full stop. You can't *choose* to lose weight from a specific body part.

Commitment: Forget about losing weight or fat from specific areas. Focus on overall health and full-body weight loss. Get into health rituals, not trouble-spots.

Long-Term Goals

- ☐
- ☐
- ☐
- ☐
- ☐
- ☐
- ☐
- ☐
- ☐

Journal...

Make Working Out Your New Compulsion

"No one is immune from addiction; it afflicts people of all ages, races, classes, and professions." – Patrick J. Kennedy

✔

✔

✔

✔

✔

✔

✔

✔

✔

☐

☐

☐

☐

☐

☐

☐

☐

☐

☐

I hope that you have never had to struggle with an addiction. If you haven't, this tip might still have something meaningful for you. As mentioned in an earlier tip, at its core, addiction is an unwillingness to be uncomfortable. But this also applies to our compulsions and cravings, even if they haven't erupted into full-blown dependency.

When you feel the urge to do something that is not good for you, consider that a good time to substitute something else. Exercise works for many people. For instance, what if, when you realized you were craving a drink, and you didn't want to give in, you went to the gym instead? Or if that wasn't convenient, that you did a quick round of exercises in your home? Or you just did a couple of pushups, or held a plank? A momentary burst of exertion will definitely take your mind off of your need for a brief time, and in some cases, maybe it's enough to get you past it.

All bad habits are vanquished by the formation of new habits. If nothing else has seemed to work for you, consider making exercise of any duration a substitute for those times of need.

Commitment: If you're struggling with a compulsion or addiction, think of something physical you could do instead.

Journal...

Keep The Things You're Trying To Avoid Out Of Your Home

"You know, all that really matters is that the people you love are happy and healthy. Everything else is just sprinkles on the sundae." – Paul Walker

To-Do's		Long-Term Goals

✔

✔

✔

✔

✔

✔

✔

It takes more effort to go to a store, or a restaurant, to buy and eat a bunch of unhealthy food, than it is to walk to your pantry to do it. It takes more effort to go to a bar and drink than to go to your refrigerator and take out a bottle of liquor. Now, going out to get yourself a treat doesn't require Herculean effort, but it does require more.

If you're trying to cut back on something, not having it in the place where you live is a great start. Once you have a plan, start getting rid of the things you want to avoid. It's not foolproof, but it will force you to make bigger choices and go out of your way to pursue your cravings. **This might call your attention to the issue sufficiently to at least make you take a breath before acting.**

Commitment: Whatever you're trying to avoid, get it out of the house, and keep it out. A poison is a poison. Why would you keep it in your house?

☐ ☐ ☐ ☐ ☐ ☐ ☐

Journal...

The Danger In Extremes

"Balance is good, because one extreme or the other leads to misery, and I've spent a lot of my life at one of those extremes." — Trent Reznor

To-Do's		Long-Term Goals

Even a state of euphoria eventually exhausts its owner. Rock bottom misery is obviously not something we want. For some patients, this is the point when they decide to do something about their obesity. But zealotry in any area tends to produce one of these two extremes. Zealotry and dogma are the realms of "always" and "never." Speaking in absolutes even though we are limited in our knowledge.

Happiness is not found in the extremes, because **extremes are tenuous, unsustainable states, fleeting and on-the-fringe by their very natures.** Even the excitement of weight loss surgery soon dissipates. Contentment is not found at the far flung poles of various issues and stances.

Be passionate, but watch yourself. If any areas of your life seem to suffer because you are being consumed by a cause or view or action, it may be time to take a hard look at things.

Commitment: Avoid extremes. Check in with yourself periodically to evaluate your viewpoints and your motivations for holding them. The key to success is consistency, not extremes.

Journal...

Don't Get Trapped By A Lifestyle

"If you're not clipping coupons before going to the grocery store, you're overspending. If you're ordering in or going out to dinner because you don't feel like cooking, you're overspending. If you're not tracking where your money is going, you're very likely overspending." – Jean Chatzky

To-Do's
✓
✓
✓
✓
✓
✓
✓
✓
✓

Long-Term Goals

☐ ☐ ☐ ☐ ☐ ☐ ☐ ☐ ☐ ☐

In the movie *Cinderella Man,* which is set during The Great Depression, there's a scene where someone visits the home of the character played by Paul Giamatti. He's a boxing promoter who has to keep up appearances. When we go through the opulent-looking door of what seems like it will be a lavish apartment, it's startling to see that it's almost completely unfurnished inside. He has to keep up appearances, you see.

But we don't need an example this extreme to know that **we can trap ourselves in a lifestyle with our spending habits.** If you make enough money to buy a fancy car and a big house, but can just barely make the payments, and can't save any money, you're going to be in trouble someday, whether you're making $500,000 a year, or $50,000.

But there's an easy way to go about living within your means. Ask if you can save money each time you get paid. If not, you're asking for problems. Do you *need* the new car? Do you *need* the bigger house? What is your peace of mind worth to you?

Commitment: Save money. Don't buy too much. Live and plan as if you will one day have to spend a few months unemployed. A better option than saving is to increase your income but then don't spend the extra income.

Journal...

Wear Your Seatbelt

"Even in the limo, I buckle my seatbelt. I got that seatbelt on before the car moves." – Christopher Walken

To-Do's

✔

✔

✔

✔

✔

Long-Term Goals

☐

☐

☐

☐

☐

Olympic Lifting coach Dan John is often asked about the minute details of various programs and lifts. His response is usually, "Do you wear your seatbelt and floss your teeth?" If the answer is no, he says, "Then I don't have any reason to think I can expect you to remember the details of a program or lift.

Which brings us to what is probably the shortest tip in this book. Driving or riding, wear your seatbelt. There is literally no excuse not to do it. This small act has saved countless lives.

Commitment: Wear your seatbelt. 100% of the time. Even in the backseat.

Journal...

DIY Videos

"Tell me and I forget. Teach me and I remember. Involve me and I learn." – Benjamin Franklin

To-Do's		Long-Term Goals

✔

✔

✔

✔

✔

✔

✔

With the information available on the Internet, it feels like you can learn anything. From knot-tying to pet grooming to the blueprints for submarine engines, you can find just about anything you can type into a search engine. But not every subject has tutorials written out.

Moreover, learning something like tying a bow tie or anything else that requires multiple steps of moderate dexterity, *watching* it can be even more effective. But it doesn't even have to be something physical. There are now tutorials on Youtube of just about anything, from publishing a blog post to grammar training. It's worth a try.

So if you're looking for something and you can't find an article about it, don't forget about video. **Think of YouTube as a search engine for videos.**

Commitment: Go to Youtube and type in "Useful DIY skills." You might be surprised at just how much there is.

☐ ☐ ☐ ☐ ☐ ☐ ☐

Journal...

No Excuses

"No excuses and no sob stories. Life is full of excuses if you're looking. I have no time to gripe over misfortune. I don't waste time looking back." – Junior Seau

To-Do's
✔
✔
✔
✔
✔
✔

There are always reasons why things don't go right, and why plans change. Legitimate reasons. And these are not excuses. Excuses are when we *do* have responsibility for something and we say that it was out of our control, or we blame someone else for it.

Excuses are when we say "I wish I was reading more books!" after binge watching an entire season of Netflix over a weekend, acting like it couldn't possibly have gone another way. Excuses are when we say that we don't have time to exercise, but we have time to play another round of Candy Crush on the iPhone.

Commitment: No more excuses. You will make mistakes. Plans will change. Just own it and keep moving. Success is found in daily rituals.

Long-Term Goals

☐
☐
☐
☐
☐
☐

Journal...

Compete!

"Competition gives me energy. It keeps me focused." – Conor McGregor

To-Do's		Long-Term Goals

✔

✔

✔

✔

✔

✔

✔

✔

✔

✔

It's never too late to enter a competition. For this tip, it doesn't even matter what kind of competition it is. You don't have to sign up for a marathon, or a bodybuilding show, or sit down across from a chess master in a tournament. But first, let's talk about why competition can be so useful and enjoyable.

First and foremost, if you're not a regular competitor, **a competition can be the perfect opportunity to work on a *specific* goal.** If your training has been lacking motivation, knowing that you're going to have to compete soon can help you focus and stay fired up. The fact that you'll have to show your skills, or strength, or whatever, in front of an audience or crowd can work wonders for your intensity.

Do a quick web search for competitions in your area. Don't just think physical, like running, swimming, or cycling. Think also artistic, like painting, music, or ballroomdance. See what's available. The range of categories might surprise you.

Commitment: Find a competition that you would enjoy and sign up for it. Don't worry about winning, or even excelling, just focus on improving.

Journal...

You Against You

"Always be yourself, express yourself, have faith in yourself. Do not go out and look for a successful personality and duplicate it." – Bruce Lee

To-Do's		Long-Term Goals
✔	The easiest way to make progress is to ignore the progress of others. If you want to be stronger, you will inevitably come across people stronger than you. If you want to run faster, you will run into people whose top times in the 400m dash will smoke you, no matter how hard you work. This applies to any art or craft or discipline or aesthetic category we could come up with.	☐
✔		☐
✔		☐
✔	And when it happens, you will be tempted to compare your results to theirs. But the only thing that any of us should worry about is whether we are better than we were yesterday. Are we stronger? Smarter? Healthier? Slimmer? Better-read?	☐
✔		☐
✔	These are the things we can control. You against you. Me against me. This was Michael Jordan's credo. **And the best part is, these are the battles that can *always* be won, and the results that can always be improved.**	☐
✔		☐
✔	**Commitment:** Tell yourself that it is you against you, and ignore the rest of the noise. Now go outdo yourself, even if just by a little bit, and celebrate yourself for it.	☐

Journal...

No Phone In The Car

"My life has been a whole series of accidents, some of them happy, some not." – Randy Bachman

To-Do's
✔
✔
✔
✔
✔
✔
✔
✔

This is very simple. The chances of you *needing* to reach for your phone while driving are very slim. The chances of you *wanting* to reach for your phone are higher, if you're like most people. Talking on your phone while driving is distracting enough. I hope it doesn't even need to be said that texting—either reading or sending—while behind the wheel is absolute madness.

Think about what driving a car actually means. It is thousands upon thousands of micro-decisions that all require your attention. Not to mention that you're sharing the road with other drivers who better all be doing the same thing. Driving can go so wrong, so quickly. There is no reason to divide your attention.

If your phone rings and you must answer it, pull over to the shoulder. The end.

Commitment: Do not talk or text on the phone while driving. Save that response for when you've arrived at your destination.

Long-Term Goals
☐
☐
☐
☐
☐
☐
☐
☐

Journal...

Go Vegan For a Month

"The best part of being a vegan is the purity and peace of mind one experiences and the strong connection I feel to the animal kingdom." – Uri Geller

To-Do's		Long-Term Goals

The commitment it takes to eat a vegan—or even vegetarian—diet can seem baffling to people who don't do it or have never tried it. If you need a primer, here's the breakdown: Vegans do not eat anything that contains or is derived from animal products. Eggs, cheese, meat, fish, and more. Vegetarians do not eat meat. That's the least you need to know about each group.

Some do it for health reasons, and some do it as a political and ethical action to protest the abominable conditions of factory farming. But whatever the reasons, and regardless of the debates surrounding whether these choices are right or wrong, there is one indisputable truth: **eating vegan has a beneficial effect on the body.** There are plenty of studies that "prove" and "disprove" nearly any claim you may have heard about these diets, for better or worse. But it is such a radical change to most people's diets that there is no way it could *not* have an affect.

Commitment: Do enough research to know how to supplement your needs. Then, if you're curious, switch to a vegan diet for a month. Learn about a vegan lifestyle, which is a level beyond just the vegan diet.

Journal...

Learn How To Feel Your Muscles

"Paying attention and awareness are universal capacities of human beings." – Jon Kabat-Zinn

To-Do's		Long-Term Goals

✔

✔

✔

✔

✔

✔

✔

✔

✔

✔

If your goal is to put more muscle on your frame, whether it's 5 pounds or 50, you have to subject your various muscles to stress. There are always ways to do this more effectively, but few will be as helpful as knowing how to *feel* each muscle that you're working. This is often called the "mind-muscle connection."

For instance, you know that doing squats "Works your legs." But can you slow down and feel it in your quadriceps? Do you know when your triceps—the three-headed muscle on the back of your arms—is working? If not, it's harder to gauge whether the exercises you're doing for those muscles are working as well as they could.

The easiest way to learn how to feel each muscle is to learn how to flex each muscle. This doesn't mean you need to spend an hour a day in front of the mirror, posing and purple-faced with effort. **But when you lift, slow down and pay attention to what's happening in your body.** Don't just think about moving the weight, notice where the body is being stressed. When you put the weight down, see if you can reproduce the effect by flexing that muscle.

Commitment: Learn how to flex each muscle. When doing your exercises, mentally focus on that particular muscle group.

Journal...

_____
_____
_____
_____
_____
_____
_____
_____
_____
_____
_____
_____
_____
_____
_____
_____
_____
_____
_____

The Delayed Gratification Method

"Delayed gratification is a sweet lesson whose teacher knows the best is not right now, it is yet to be." –
Maximillian Degenerez

To-Do's		Long-Term Goals

I once heard someone say that people were as easy to train as dogs. I'm not sure that person had ever had a dog, but there was something to his reasoning. Our brains are pattern-making machines. We teach them and they react. Teach the same thing enough times, and the brain then expects the same result in the same situation.

This is wonderful if the habits are good. If they're bad, you've now set yourself a tougher hill to climb. Enter the delayed gratification method, which is so simple that it barely feels like a method at all.

1. Ask yourself "What's the right thing for me to be doing?" (Right, as in, for your goals)

2. How will I reward myself for doing it? (come up with an appropriate reward)

3. If you do the right thing, reward yourself. If not, withhold it.

It doesn't get any simpler than that. But we're not always great at delaying our gratification. Try this simple method. If it works, you know you're serious about your goals. If it doesn't, then you've learned something about priorities.

Commitment: Practice the delayed gratification method.

Journal...

Muscle Burns Fat—Get Some

"You really have to have some muscle to be on the stage in front of the world." – Billy Crystal

To-Do's		Long-Term Goals

The last thing many people want to do when they're trying to lose weight is to add muscle to their frame. It makes sense, but only because they're thinking too much about the number on the scale. The truth is that a body with more muscle is a more efficient fat-burning machine. **Muscle burns fat.**

Dani Shugart from *T Nation* puts it this way: *Don't think of muscle as more weight on the scale or more size on your frame. Think of it as metabolically expensive tissue that will help you get leaner and eventually lose a lot of fat.* If you have more muscle, you can also eat more while avoiding the normal repercussions of a caloric surplus.

You'll also have a stronger, healthier body with more aesthetic appeal. There are no downsides to gaining some muscle, whatever your goals are. No one starts lifting and suddenly explodes into a regrettable pile of muscle. Put on a few lean pounds and watch the change.

Commitment: Gain a few pounds of muscle. Watch your waistline drop. As you get older, it is imperative that you maintain your lean muscle.

Journal...

November 27

Every Body Is Different

"If any thing is sacred, the human body is sacred." – Walt Whitman

To-Do's

✔

✔

✔

✔

✔

✔

✔

✔

Long-Term Goals

For all that we've talked about not comparing ourselves to others, there's one area where it can be truly, physically unhealthy. About the worst thing you can do is to look at someone with horrible eating habits, but who also has a good physique, and model your eating after theirs. "Well, so and so does it and he/she looks healthy, so…"

Every body is different. **Every metabolism works a little differently at every age.** Some people have genetics that mean, at least for a while, they can seemingly eat whatever they want and not add an ounce of fat. Some people are on performance enhancing drugs that mean they can cut a few corners. But we all know what unhealthy eating looks like, and the fact that someone who looks good is eating like a kid in a candy store doesn't mean they're a good nutritional model.

Commitment: Stick to what you know. Nutrition is pretty simple. Avoid the temptation to eat like someone else just because it seems to work for them.

☐ ☐ ☐ ☐ ☐ ☐ ☐ ☐

Journal...

Don't Copy The Routines Of The Pros

"It's hard work to find your own voice and not to copycat anything." – Arnaud Desplechin

To-Do's

- ✓
- ✓
- ✓
- ✓
- ✓
- ✓
- ✓
- ✓
- ✓
- ✓

Long-Term Goals

- ☐
- ☐
- ☐
- ☐
- ☐
- ☐
- ☐
- ☐
- ☐

When you are resolving to get back into the habit of whatever your version of fitness is—bodybuilding, running, Crossfit, swimming, etc.—it's natural to start scanning the web for articles about what you "should" do. And you will inevitably come across the routines of champions and professionals that purport to tell you exactly how to look/perform like them.

The problem is that the gap between their abilities and those of the average person who just wants to get back in shape again is vast, and attaining their results is most likely unattainable. Genetics matter. Training matters. **The amount of years they have spent honing their skills or physiques matter.** To say nothing of the possibility that maybe *they* aren't using the routines listed in web articles or magazines. Or that they didn't use them to get where they are today.

Go into a new program with your eyes open. The basics always work, and the basics never comprise the program of someone performing at an elite level.

Commitment: Do not blindly copy the routines of the pros. Find out what works for *you*. Find something you enjoy doing and keep doing it.

Journal...

Pay In Cash

"Number one...cash is king." – Jack Welch

To-Do's
✔
✔
✔
✔
✔
✔
✔
✔
✔

Long-Term Goals

☐
☐
☐
☐
☐
☐
☐
☐
☐

Credit cards can seem like magic money. Or worse, like they don't involve money at all. The debit to your card can just feel like it's numbers on a screen out there somewhere, happening to someone else. When you look at your account, you see the change, but it's easy to put off looking at an account if you're not in the mood to see the numbers going down.

Cash is different. You have to take it out to pay for something. Then, there's less of it than before, and **you can see it** in real time. It is a visual choice. If you can get yourself on a cash budget, then you may find that your money goes further because you have to watch yourself part with it, transaction by transaction.

Obviously, you want to be wise about it. Carrying around a thousand bucks in cash is going to sting more if you lose your wallet than if you were carrying a twenty. But whenever possible, try carrying cash and see if it makes you more frugal or thoughtful.

Commitment: Commit to a month of primarily cash transactions. Give yourself a weekly cash budget and spend only the cash you have in your wallet for that week.

Journal...

Protect Your Ears

"Men trust their ears less than their eyes." – Herodotus

To-Do's

- ✔
- ✔
- ✔
- ✔
- ✔
- ✔
- ✔
- ✔
- ✔

Long-Term Goals

- ☐
- ☐
- ☐
- ☐
- ☐
- ☐
- ☐
- ☐
- ☐

Youth conveys a sense of indestructibility on those lucky enough—and naive enough—to be caught in its throes. Behaviors that might send your 35-year-old self into anxious convulsions might be laughed off. Sure, I'll jump off the bridge. I'll drive down this road backwards. I can drink a whole fifth of whiskey, etc. But the examples don't have to be extreme to be valid.

Hearing loss, and its prevention, probably sounds lamer than anything to a kid. But if you're an adult whose hearing is as good as it was when you were 15, you're probably in the minority. Concerts, backfiring cars, band practice, gunfire for the hunters and sport shooters, and more, can do irreparable damage to our ears in later life.

When you know something's going to be loud, learning to plug your ears when you're young—and continuing to do so when you're older—is an easy habit, and an important one. If you're going into a prolonged situation at high volume, there's nothing wrong with wearing earplugs.

Commitment: Protect your hearing whenever you can. Make it a habit. This includes earbuds.

Journal...

December

Avoid Over-Indulging During The Holidays

"All holidays can be good times." – John Clayton

To-Do's		Long-Term Goals

If you're in a country where Christmas is celebrated, the next 31 days may be a challenge to your fitness resolutions. The holidays are a time to enjoy good food and have a blast, but you can do that and *still* not jettison all of your plans and goals. We don't *need* to eat candy every day, even if someone brings it into work every day. Even if you love the seasonal toffee at the grocery store you don't have a *duty* to buy it and eat it.

Instead, practice moderation in your food choices, and consider increasing the intensity and/or frequency of your exercise during December. If you binge one night, eat a few hours later than usual the next morning, just to give your body a longer fasted state. **Don't beat yourself up if you mess up.** You probably will. Maybe you *should*. It's neither holly nor jolly to be at a Christmas party and not touch any of the food.

Be smart. Celebrate. Control what you can.

Commitment: Make this the healthiest December you've ever had.

Journal...

December 2

Start Your Resolutions Now

"I think in terms of the day's resolutions, not the year's." – Henry Moore

To-Do's
✔
✔
✔
✔
✔
✔
✔

New Year's Day is coming up, and that can make it easy to indulge throughout December, because, well, New Year's resolutions are coming as well. But think about what this means. Do any of us really need a day, a specific *day,* to set new goals and do better? And if you're like most of us, you've probably had the joy of seeing your New Year's resolutions fade or outright implode by February.

I'd like to suggest an alternative. **Be the kind of driven person who does not need to make resolutions for the year, because you are already pursuing the things that matter to you, every day.** These are not things that require resolve, or huge changes, but rather, they are a cascade of the small, good habits that results in happiness, health, and prosperity.

Commitment: Make your resolutions today and get started. Don't wait for January 1. Write them out twice a day.

Long-Term Goals

☐ ☐ ☐ ☐ ☐ ☐ ☐

Journal...

Hang Out

"A good stance and posture reflect a proper state of mind." – Morihei Ueshiba

To-Do's

- ✔
- ✔
- ✔
- ✔
- ✔
- ✔
- ✔

Long-Term Goals

- ☐
- ☐
- ☐
- ☐
- ☐
- ☐
- ☐

If you sit for most of the day at work, or if you exercise with heavy weights, there's a good chance that your spine is getting compressed. This is the kind of thing that's hard to notice. It's not like you wake up and realize that you're an inch shorter than you used to be because your spine is squished. **But even the micro-compressions that can be caused by poor posture add up over time.**

If you're strong enough to do it—and if you're not, it's not hard to develop the sufficient amount of strength—you can make great progress and keep your spine happier by regularly spending a few seconds hanging from something. A bar, a tree branch, whatever. Try some gravity boots. Your bodyweight and gravity will pull you down and if you can loosen up, you'll feel your spine stretch and lengthen.

Commitment: Develop the amount of strength required to hang from a bar. Do this regularly to counteract the daily demands placed on the spine.

Journal...

_____
_____
_____
_____
_____
_____
_____
_____
_____
_____
_____
_____
_____
_____
_____
_____
_____
_____
_____
_____
_____
_____
_____

Don't Go To Bed Mad

"I am a danger to myself if I get angry." – Oriani Fallaci

✔

✔

✔

✔

✔

✔

✔

☐

☐

☐

☐

☐

☐

☐

☐

This is an oldie but a goodie. Even when things are going well, sleep can be elusive. If you're busy, the moments after you get in bed might be the first time in the day when your thoughts are truly your own. This is great, unless that's when all of the stressful thoughts rush in, and now you're agitated and calming your mind now sounds like a bad joke.

But anger is even worse than the agitation of restlessness. If you go to bed angry—whether you've just had an argument, or something has happened, or you remembered something else that made you mad, etc.—it can be *really* hard to turn it off. **It's best if you can deal with the anger before you get in bed.** Zone out, make up, forgive the other person, color, meditate, journal, whatever it takes to deal with whatever's happening.

Fix it before you try to sleep.

Commitment: Do not try to sleep while angry. Chances are you won't be able to. Instead, try journaling or goal setting. Refocus your anger into something more productive.

Journal...

Give Yourself A Compliment

"A compliment is something like a kiss through a veil." – Victor Hugo

To-Do's

✔

✔

✔

✔

✔

✔

✔

✔

Long-Term Goals

☐ ☐ ☐ ☐ ☐ ☐ ☐ ☐ ☐

The next time you see yourself in the mirror, pretend that it's a stranger you're looking at. Now pretend that you want to make this stranger feel good. You're going to give this person in the mirror a compliment. Now, if you don't like yourself, this exercise might make your skin crawl, but that just means that you'll get more out of this than anyone if you do it regularly.

No cheating. **Just keep looking at yourself, this stranger, until you think of something nice to say.** It can be anything, but you have to do it. It could be a compliment about the clothes you're wearing, the color of your eyes, the warmth of your smile, and so on. You can even cheat and compliment yourself on things the mirror doesn't know. You can tell yourself that you are kind, and intelligent, and funny. Anything.

But you have to do it.

Commitment: Now that you've done it, stay in the habit. Do it everytime you look into a reflective surface. One of the best ways to see yourself approvingly is to talk to yourself approvingly, whether the compliments are verbal or internal.

Journal...

Surprise People (In A Good Way)

"I don't know why it surprises people that I surprise them." – Liz Phair

To-Do's		Long-Term Goals

✔

✔

✔

✔

✔

Aside from grouches like Don Draper in *Mad Men,* it's safe to assume that plenty of people like surprises. So much of life is routine. **So much restlessness and boredom comes from the fact that sometimes *nothing* unexpected seems to happen.** A nice surprise changes that, and you can also be that surprise for someone else.

Whether it's a kind word, a small gift, a phone call to an old friend, or any of the innumerable small, sweet things we might do for another person, surprises last. Surprises are memorable. And they don't have to require much effort or cost to be meaningful.

Commitment: Try to surprise someone each day this week. Make a memory for them. And for you.

☐ ☐ ☐ ☐ ☐

Journal...

Share Your Talents

"True happiness involves the full use of one's power and talents." – John W. Gardner

To-Do's		Long-Term Goals

Think about all of the music that you love. And the movies. And the books. And the TV shows. And all of the art that's hanging on all of the walls of the world. The sculptures that are sitting on pedestals in museums. These things, and more, are all the result of people sharing their talents. Maybe they did it for passion, maybe they did it for profit, but for those of us who enjoy the art, the result is the same.

You have talents as well, even if you don't yet know what they are. **One of the surest ways for each of us to improve the world is to share our talents.** Maybe we never have a gigantic audience, but change doesn't need to happen on a massive scale in order to be meaningful.

If you're truly stuck as to what your talents might be, we've talked a lot in this book about finding passions and hobbies, and learning. There's something out there. Keep looking.

Commitment: Develop and share your talents. Even on a small scale. You'll enrich someone else's life. Who knows, you might even change the world.

Journal...

If I Could Change One Thing

"When I found out I had cancer, I just said one thing: 'I want to hold on to life' and that changed everything for me." – Scott Thompson

To-Do's
✔
✔
✔
✔
✔
✔
✔
✔

Imagine that a genie appears in front of you. He offers to change one thing about the world, and you get to pick. What would you choose? **Would it be something for yourself, or for humanity at large?** Would you ask for unimaginable wealth? Would you ask for world peace? An end to poverty or hunger?

Would you wish that everyone had something to be passionate about? Would you ask for immortality? Would you want to go back to the past and change your actions? Now, pretend the genie is making you pick, and if you don't, humanity is going to be in trouble.

Really think about this. If you could change one thing, what would it be? The answer might be a clue to what your priorities are.

Commitment: Stare down the genie and make your choice. See if you can decide what would give the world the most bang for the buck. Do you believe in yourself enough to ask for ultimate power?

Long-Term Goals

☐
☐
☐
☐
☐
☐
☐
☐

Journal...

Contemplate The Golden Rule

"I just live and let live, and live my life pretty much according to the Golden Rule. And it turns out well for me." – *Dean Cain*

To-Do's
✔
✔
✔
✔
✔
✔

The Golden Rule says to treat others the way we want to be treated. It sounds good. Maybe it is good. Right? After all, what could be more simple? What could be wrong with treating others the way that you want them to treat you?

It depends on what you think you deserve, and on how you think people should treat you. If you're a victim and you're in love with your melancholy, that is how people will see you. There is a payoff and you get something out of continuing to act like a victim. If you're a narcissist, you think the world revolves around you.

What's better? Treating people the way *they* want to be treated. This requires listening and effort, and doesn't have anything to do with what we each think we deserve.

Commitment: Treat people how they want to be treated. Much of the world knows this rule but chooses to ignore it.

Long-Term Goals
☐
☐
☐
☐
☐
☐

Journal...

Take A Vacation Without a Schedule

"A vacation spot out of season always has a very special magic." – Max Von Sydow

To-Do's		Long-Term Goals

The benefits of taking a vacation are many and obvious. However, free time and vacation days are not there in an endless supply. So you can wind up packing so much into a vacation that you return home more exhausted than when you left. These types of vacations usually revolve around specific locations and touristy attractions.

But a vacation doesn't have to have a detailed itinerary. **One way to ensure that you get to do some relaxing is to take an open-ended vacation.** For instance, take a road trip with the understanding that you'll stop along the way and do or see anything that looks interesting. You'll be free to let your mood and your company dictate the pace of the trip, and how you spend the time.

Hopefully, when you're back, you'll actually feel rested and rewarded for how hard you work.

Commitment: Take a *relaxing* vacation. Ditch the itinerary unless you absolutely hate the thought of it.

Journal...

Ask For Help

"We are all here on earth to help others; what on earth the others are here for I don't know." – W.H. Auden

To-Do's
✔
✔
✔
✔
✔
✔
✔
✔
✔

Long-Term Goals

☐ ☐ ☐ ☐ ☐ ☐ ☐ ☐ ☐

Sometimes pride can keep us from healing, or progressing, or forgiving. There are going to be times when we simply can't solve our own problems. We will need to be able to rely on other people. People who we can ask for help, if we're willing to.

When you are hurting, are you able to ask for help? Do you worry about seeming weak? Do you beat yourself up because you think you should be able to make things better on your own? Think about a time when someone came to you for help. You probably didn't roll your eyes and think "Oh, what a weakling!" And the chances of someone doing that to you in a time of need are small.

The key to asking for help appropriately is to do it without any sense of entitlement. You are not *owed* anyone's help. Obviously, this does not apply if you're a kid going to your parents. They do owe you whatever support they can give you. But if you have a hard time asking for help, it's time to get over it. **You can't be your best without the help of others.** Not every time.

Commitment: Ask someone you trust for help if you need it. Let go of the idea that it's weak or needy to do so.

Journal...

_____
_____
_____
_____
_____
_____
_____
_____
_____
_____
_____
_____
_____
_____
_____
_____
_____
_____
_____
_____

Experiment With Music At The Gym

"It's nice to create something you believe in. It's even nicer to dance to your own tunes sometimes." – Shreya Ghoshal

To-Do's		Long-Term Goals

✔

✔

✔

✔

✔

✔

If you go to a public gym, there's probably music playing. And unless you have the most mainstream, poppy taste, it might not be music you can enjoy. It's easier than ever to bring your own, though, this being the age of the smartphone and iPod. You might have something you love to listen to during your workouts. But it's worth experimenting to see if there are styles of music, or tempos, that seem to boost your workouts even more.

Some people claim that music distracts them when they're really trying to concentrate during a workout. Others swear by it and can't imagine training without their tunes.

There is so much music out there. Keep experimenting.

Commitment: Don't get stuck in a rut with the music you listen to while training. Change it up and see if anything surprises you.

☐ ☐ ☐ ☐ ☐ ☐

Journal...

Consider Getting A Tailor

"A gentleman never talks about his tailor." – Nick Cave

To-Do's
✔
✔
✔
✔
✔
✔
✔
✔

You will feel better if you look better, and part of that includes how you dress. But no matter how nice your clothes are, they'll look even better if they fit correctly. "Try before you buy" is good advice, but body types are all different, and just about any garment can still be made to fit better, no matter how good it looks right off the rack.

The answer is tailoring. This doesn't mean you have to go around in bespoke suits or custom dresses. Only that a good tailor—and this doesn't have to mean expensive modifications—can take a garment and shape it to your body. Clothes are designed for the average body type, with metrics including everything from torso length to height and weight. **But there can be so much more.** Shoulder widths and waistlines can vary wildly between three people who are all the same height. So can arm length, neck thickness, back width, and so on.

Clothes can make you more confident in how you look. Tailored clothes take it one step further.

Commitment: Find a tailor you like and go through one round of alterations on your favorite items of clothing.

Long-Term Goals
☐
☐
☐
☐
☐
☐
☐
☐
☐

Journal...

Personal Grooming

"You are your greatest asset. Put your time, effort and money into training, grooming, and encouraging your greatest asset." – Tom Hopkins

To-Do's	
✔	
✔	
✔	
✔	
✔	
✔	
✔	
✔	

Long-Term Goals

☐
☐
☐
☐
☐
☐
☐
☐

Getting regular haircuts, exfoliating your skin, keeping your fingernails trim and clean, shaving often and well, and keeping your clothes neat and tidy can look obsessive to people who don't prioritize personal grooming. It can be even worse if you're a man. For some, these simple acts of self-care and self-respect seem downright unmasculine.

But there is nothing wrong with taking pride in how you look. If you had a sports car, few people who take issue with the fact that you waxed it and washed it regularly, and paid for detailing a couple of times a month. After all, the car was expensive, why wouldn't you want it to look as presentable, and run as well, as possible?

Taking care of your personal grooming is a matter of pride. It says, "I care about myself this much and want to show my best self to the world."

Commitment: If you don't have one, develop a regular grooming regimen. You'll look better, and you'll probably feel better as a result.

Journal...

Eat Before You Work Out

"I love that feeling of just finishing a workout and knowing I'm taking care of my body. It is such a good feeling."
– Jenna Ushkowitz

To-Do's		Long-Term Goals

Fasted training has its advocates. You'll often hear that working out first thing in the morning, on an empty stomach, will yield better fat-burning results than training after eating. And it might be. But ask yourself this: what is the purpose of your workout? Do you believe you will get better results if you can work out longer, and with more energy?

If you can answer yes to either of those questions, then working out in a fasted state might work against your long term goals. You will burn more calories if you can work out at greater intensities. You will also build more muscle, which then burns more fat, if you can work out with more energy. Energy comes from fuel. Food is that fuel.

The only thing you owe yourself is better results. So if you're a diehard fasted-training person, at least give yourself a chance to experience a workout with food in your stomach.

Commitment: Spend a week eating a small meal an hour or two before your workout. Make sure it contains protein and some starchy carbs. If your workouts go better—you'll know if you're tracking progress, as you should—keep going. I have a ketogenic supplement for burning fat while increasing muscle. Check it out at ducvuong.pruvitnow.com

Journal...

Train To Failure Occasionally

"If you're not failing every now and again, it's a sign you're not doing anything very innovative." – Woody Allen

To-Do's		Long-Term Goals

Have you ever heard the phrase "Train to failure" in the gym and wondered what it meant? Let's use the biceps curl as an example. Training to failure in one set would mean doing curls until you literally could not do another. In other words, muscular failure.

Now, why would you do this? The answer depends on your goals, but we can generalize a little. Even though we've talked about "no pain, no gain," being a backwards approach to health, there is great value in the occasional test of working very, very hard in the gym. If you have trained a muscle to failure, you *know* you have worked it hard. This can result in greater stimulus and hypertrophy (muscle growth) while teaching your body what it feels like to work hard.

There is no reason to go to failure on every set. **Indeed, it can be too taxing on the nervous system and impede recovery.** It also doesn't need to be done with heavy weights. Any amount of weight can be lifted until it can't be lifted anymore.

Commitment: Over your next five workouts, take five different exercises to failure during one set. See how your muscles respond during recovery.

Journal...

_____
_____
_____
_____
_____
_____
_____
_____
_____
_____
_____
_____
_____
_____
_____
_____
_____
_____
_____
_____

Take Your Body Measurements For Better Progress

"Many churches are measuring the wrong things. We measure things like attendance and giving, but we should be looking at more fundamental things like anger, contempt, honesty, and the degree to which people are under the thumb of their lusts. Those things can be counted, but not as easily as offerings." – Dallas Willard

To-Do's
✔
✔
✔
✔
✔
✔
✔
✔

"I want to be more muscular" is a goal. So is "I want to lose weight." But, "I want to put an inch on my arms," or "I want to lose fifteen pounds," are specific goals. **Remember, whatever can be measured, can be improved without guesswork.** So, if you're trying to alter your body in specific ways, you have to start out by measuring.

Have someone help you with a tape measure. Measure your neck, shoulder width, biceps circumference, chest, waist, thighs, and calves. Record the measurements in a journal. If you're trying to grow more muscular, give the areas under development some extra attention. Measure again in three weeks. If you're trying to slim down, make sure your nutrition is on point, and also measure every two to three weeks.

This is the surest way to *know* that you are getting larger or smaller, depending on your goals.

Commitment: Take your body measurements. As scary as this might be. No more guessing. See the damage the Holidays might inflict.

Long-Term Goals
☐
☐
☐
☐
☐
☐
☐
☐

Journal...

Stop Talking About What You've Done

"The beauty of the past belongs to the past." – Margaret Bourke-White

To-Do's

- ✔
- ✔
- ✔
- ✔
- ✔
- ✔
- ✔

Long-Term Goals

- ☐
- ☐
- ☐
- ☐
- ☐
- ☐
- ☐

One of the bittersweet things about the "glory days" of the past is that they're, well, in the past. Not that there's anything wrong with fond memories of achievements and accolades. However, if you're talking constantly about the victories of the past solely because the present is not a source of inspiration or pleasure, things could be better.

Remember the past with joy, but do things *now*. **Tell yourself that your best is yet to come, and then *show yourself* that it's true.** Something you wrote, or did, or ate, or caught at the last second to win the big game, does not need to be your crowning achievement.

Be proud of what you've done. Be prouder of what you are doing.

Commitment: Bring your past winning streak into the present. Do something worth talking about. Something that will be a perfect memory in the future.

Journal...

Add A Home Gym

"I actually have never been to a gym. I haven't had time. I have been working for the last 25 years. I just don't have time to put on a little outfit and go to the gym and work out and clean up and come home." – Suzanne Somers

To-Do's
✔
✔
✔
✔
✔
✔
✔
✔
✔

Even if you love the buzz of going to the gym and you never miss a workout, there are going to be times when getting there will be inconvenient or impossible. If you still have time to train, but not time to get there, adding a basic home gym can make a huge difference, because you'll never be caught without some equipment.

A home gym doesn't have to be elaborate to be effective. Someone who enjoys full body workouts can make huge progress with a squat rack and a bench press. But if space is an issue, even having a few dumbbells or kettlebells in the basement or garage takes away the excuse to not train.

And of course, we don't even need to go that far. You can *always* do some pushups or jumping jacks and other bodyweight exercises at home, even if you don't have a single piece of equipment beyond your body. Try isometric exercises.

Commitment: Add a basic home gym so that you'll always be able to exercise when you want to, and when it's inconvenient to hit the gym. Learn about isometric exercises.

Long-Term Goals
☐
☐
☐
☐
☐
☐
☐
☐
☐

Journal...

_____

_____

_____

_____

_____

_____

_____

_____

_____

_____

_____

_____

_____

_____

_____

_____

_____

_____

_____

Have At Least One Big-Ass Long Term Goal

"Audacity, more audacity, always audacity." – Georges Jacques Danton

To-Do's		Long-Term Goals
✔		☐
✔		☐
✔		☐
✔		☐
✔		☐
✔		☐
✔		☐
✔		☐

We've talked a lot about many small steps leading to great progress, and how big goals must be chopped into many, many small goals. But we haven't yet talked about goals that are massive and audacious. Goals that might take decades to achieve. It can be a lot of fun to work towards something that seems unachievable, just to see what you can make yourself do.

Say you want to see every country in the world by the time you're 70. Or you want to have a million dollars in the bank. Maybe you want to run for political office or become a CEO, or start a Fortune 500 company. Maybe you want to win an Oscar or release a bestselling album. This is Shooting For The Stars. These are goals that may prove to be unattainable, but they require such intense focus and devotion, over many years, **that there are many lessons to be learned in the mere pursuit of them.**

Commitment: Make a huge, huge goal. You don't even have to tell anyone about it. Write it down twice a day. Start taking steps toward it. Don't stop dreaming.

Journal...

_____
_____
_____
_____
_____
_____
_____
_____
_____
_____
_____
_____
_____
_____
_____
_____
_____
_____
_____
_____
_____
_____
_____

Be Your Own Hero

"A hero is somebody who is selfless, who is generous in spirit, who just tries to give back as much as possible and help people. A hero to me is someone who saves people and who really deeply cares." – Debi Mazar

To-Do's		Long-Term Goals
✔	Did you look up to any superheros when you were young? There has been such a glut of superhero movies over the past few years—with no end in sight—that it seems like Hollywood thinks most of us are looking for a hero to save us, or at least to look up to.	☐
✔		☐
✔	What if you were the hero? **What if you were the only one you had to look up to?** How would you change your life? Better yet, what if someone told you that you were going to be their son's or daughter's hero, no matter what? How might you change your behavior? Your way of thinking?	☐
✔		☐
✔	What if you *knew* that someone was going to use you for an example, no matter what?	☐
✔	**Commitment:** Shape your life so that you can be the hero of your own story. Be someone you can look up to. Do something courageous.	☐

Journal...

Write A Fan Letter

"My fan mail is what keeps me going." – Lil Kim

To-Do's

- ✓
- ✓
- ✓
- ✓
- ✓
- ✓
- ✓
- ✓

Long-Term Goals

- ☐
- ☐
- ☐
- ☐
- ☐
- ☐
- ☐
- ☐

You're never too old to admire a great musician, writer, athlete, or actor. Of course, the greats hear it all the time from their fans, but I have a hard time believing that any of them get tired of it, even though the time they can dedicate to responding to fan mail can be limited.

But it's a thrill to get a response from someone you admire. With social media, the barriers to connecting are lower than they've ever been. Lebron James might never read your letter, but the chances that he sees a comment left on his Twitter are much higher. Not that you need to run and sign up for Twitter.

Writing a heartfelt letter of appreciation to someone whose work has enriched your life can also help you articulate just how meaningful they have been for you. And it may inspire you to start over with their entire body of work. And remember, there's always a chance that you *will* get a response.

Commitment: Write a fan letter to someone you love and admire. It does not need to be a celebrity.

Journal...

Write A Mission Statement

"A man with money is no match against a man on a mission." – Doyle Brunson

To-Do's

✔

✔

✔

✔

✔

✔

✔

✔

✔

If you work in an office, the company you work for might have a mission statement. It's a clarification of the goals and values of the organization, and is ostensibly the plan against which all employees will measure their performance, decisions, and output.

For instance, here is IKEA's Mission Statement: *At IKEA our vision is to create a better everyday life for many people. Our business idea supports this vision by offering a wide range of well-designed, functional home furnishing products at prices so low that as many people as possible will be able to afford them.* Nothing hard to understand about that, right?

Now, what would your own mission statement look like? **It would require you to know your purpose and to have a strategy.** A mission statement is like a beacon in the night, which keeps you on the right path and signals the need for course corrections.

Commitment: Write your own mission statement for your life. Make it grand in scope but succinct in verbiage. Read it often.

Long-Term Goals

☐

☐

☐

☐

☐

☐

☐

☐

☐

Journal...

Take Time For Devotion

"How we pay attention to the present moment largely determines the character of our experience and, therefore, the quality of our lives" – Sam Harris

To-Do's		**Long-Term Goals**

We get better at whatever we do. If sitting still for one minute in quiet contemplation feels like a fidgety eternity to you, then this is a clear sign that calm reflection is not something you experience often.

If you are a spiritual and/or religious person, your chances to commune with your idea of divinity will scale with your ability to sit still and focus. If you are an open-minded seeker, the solace of solitude will enhance your ability to search. If you are a skeptic, or even hostile to the idea of spirituality, there are still benefits to be had from the practice of devotion, which can look like prayer, meditation, guided breathing, a moment of silence, and so on.

We don't need to get so grand in scope to make the case for tranquil introspection. On a smaller scale, when life feels like a fire drill, or when your day feels like nothing but a relentless series of tasks to be accomplished before you collapse onto your bed, how much can you really be enjoying things? **Real joy comes from being present.** Being present depends on how thoughtful we can be. And that depends on how often we're willing to practice devotion.

Commitment: Every day, starting with today, turn your attention to your breathing for five minutes. If you prefer to think during this time, think only of the good things in your life. Verbalize 5 things that you are grateful for in your life.

Journal...

Contemplate Your Place In This Universe

"To the mind that is still, the whole universe surrenders." – Lao Tzu

To-Do's		Long-Term Goals

Christmas is a day of contemplation and thanks for Christians. Despite the commercialization of the holiday, it is still a day when millions upon millions of people turn their thoughts to their most sacred beliefs, regardless of their religious affiliations. And you don't have to be a believer to do it today.

Spend some time today thinking about your most deeply-held beliefs. Are you a person of faith? Do you believe in an afterlife? Reaffirm your commitments as you head into the new year. Or, are you a skeptic? An atheist? An agnostic? Do you believe that we are all alone, whirling through space on our little planet? No more than blips on the cosmic timeline? How do you feel about this? Again, just think it through.

This is a wonderful day to write down the reasons for your faith, or lack of it. **There is comfort in both, depending on your perspective.**

Commitment: Take today to contemplate your place, or lack of it, in whatever you consider the Big Picture to be.

Journal...

Be Reliable

"Being taken for granted is an unpleasant but sincere form of praise. Ironically, the more reliable you are, and the less you complain, the more likely you are to be taken for granted." – Gretchen Rubin

To-Do's		Long-Term Goals

When you say that you'll do something, or be somewhere, do the people closest to you believe it? Do you have a habit of being unreliable with the people who will always forgive you? If so, now's the time to change it. We are only as good as our word, **even if we are forgiven for our carelessness.**

Honestly, if you were always inconvenienced by an unreliable person, you'd want them to change it, right? And you'd probably think that changing it was within their power. This isn't rocket science. Well, if you can believe that, then it's not a stretch to suggest that you wouldn't want someone else to feel that way about you.

Commitment: Be reliable. Do what you say you'll do. Be where you say you'll be. Take pride in knowing that people can depend on you.

✔
✔
✔
✔
✔
✔

☐
☐
☐
☐
☐
☐

Journal...

"That's Just The Way I Am"

"All habits gather unseen degrees, as brooks make rivers, rivers run to seas." – John Dryden

To-Do's		Long-Term Goals

✔

✔

✔

✔

✔

✔

✔

✔

✔

"Oh, I just have a temper." "I'm stubborn." "I always have to have the last word." "I'm a worrier." "I'm just a shy person." I could go on all day, but here's the point. We all have ideas about who we are and what we are like. There is definitely something to be said for the fact that we're all wired a little differently. However, acknowledging this can also open the door to excuses.

Do I really *know* that I'm stubborn, and that I can never change? It's a convenient thought. If I *know* I can never change, then I don't have to try, do I? Once I know "what I'm like," then I can let myself off the hook. If other people can't deal with my quirks, that's their responsibility, yes? Maybe. But maybe not.

Whatever you think you know about yourself, take another look. **There are always behaviors that we can change.** It would be easier not to. It would be natural not to. But this is responsibility shifting, and it allows us to perpetuate behaviors that we would not condone in others.

Commitment: Let go of "That's just the way I am" and continue looking for ways to be better. Improving in one small aspect of your personality would be a great way to end the year!

☐ ☐ ☐ ☐ ☐ ☐ ☐ ☐ ☐

Journal...

Use The Winter To Gain A Little Weight

"In winter, I plot and plan. In spring, I move." – Henry Rollins

To-Do's

- ✔
- ✔
- ✔
- ✔
- ✔
- ✔
- ✔
- ✔
- ✔
- ✔

Long-Term Goals

☐ ☐ ☐ ☐ ☐ ☐ ☐ ☐ ☐ ☐

If you look at bodybuilding magazines around this time of year, there are a lot of articles about "winter bulking." If you live in a cold climate that requires you to cover up, those articles are usually aimed at you. They say that now is the time to gain weight because you'll be covered up by sweaters and coats for the rest of the season and no one will know you've picked up some extra weight.

Bodybuilders often do this because bulking up leads to increased body mass. Some of it will be muscle—assuming they keep training—and some of it will be fat. Then, when they shed the extra pounds for summer, they'll lose the extra fat and keep the extra muscle. There can be some validity to this, but it has to be done under control.

Too often, "bulking" becomes the excuse to eat 100 Pop Tarts for breakfast, followed by fried chicken and chips for lunch, and then a bunch of pasta and pizza for dinner. The number on the scale moved, so you gained weight! **But it shouldn't be the wrong kind of weight.** If you're going to do a mild winter bulk, simply increase your calories—which you are hopefully tracking—by 500 per week and see if you gain. There's no reason to go overboard.

Commitment: Experiment this winter and put on a few extra pounds, if that fits your goals. Train hard, increase your calories slightly, and you'll pick up some mass. You'll have plenty of time to shed any extra flab that you pick up in time for tank top season.

Journal...

Watch A Sunrise And A Sunset

"There was never a night or a problem that could defeat sunrise or hope." – Bernard Williams

To-Do's

✔

✔

✔

✔

✔

✔

✔

✔

✔

Long-Term Goals

☐

☐

☐

☐

☐

☐

☐

☐

☐

Sunrises and sunsets are a couple of the most overused items in literature. But authors compare various sorts of beauty to sunrises and sunsets because, well...they're beautiful. Clichés stick around for a reason—there's always some truth to them.

If you're not a morning person, or if you're a night owl, maybe it's been a while since you've watched a sunrise. Give yourself the experience again. If you're somewhere with mountains, the higher up you can get, the better the view will be. Or, you can just set your alarm, sit by your living room window, and see the light start to creep across the sky.

Sunrise and sunset are a great time for reflection and stillness. In the right frame of mind, it's hard not to be moved by the sight of time passing before your eyes in a burst of color, especially as another year is coming to an end.

Commitment: Choose a day when you can watch a sunrise and sunset. Write about the experience in your journal. Tomorrow night would be a great night to try for example.

Journal...

Feel Better After The Party

"Alcohol may be man's worst enemy, but the bible says love your enemy." – Frank Sinatra

To-Do's		Long-Term Goals

✔

✔

✔

✔

✔

✔

✔

✔

If you're celebrating New Year's Eve tonight, you might be in the mood to party hard. And that's fine. But there are ways to have your fun *and* not feel like a train ran over you tomorrow morning. If you're a drinker, here are a couple of tips that you can implement throughout the long evening and night that will give you a better day tomorrow.

Pace yourself. Drink one glass of water for every alcoholic drink you consume. You'll stay hydrated and still be able to retain a buzz. Also, have a good meal before you start drinking. Meaning, protein, carbs, and good fats. It will set you up for a speedier recovery in the aftermath.

You can also limit yourself to a drink per hour. Drinking five cocktails over the space of five hours has a vastly different effect on you than drinking five cocktails in two hours. **Have fun, but do your near-future self a couple of favors, and you can bring in the New Year without regrets.**

Commitment: Are you getting ready for the New Year? If you're drinking tonight, implement these tips for a better day tomorrow.

☐ ☐ ☐ ☐ ☐ ☐ ☐ ☐

Journal...

What If Today Were Your Last Day?

"I wake up every day and I think, 'I'm breathing! It's a good day.'" – Eve Ensler

To-Do's
✔
✔
✔
✔
✔
✔
✔

Long-Term Goals
☐
☐
☐
☐
☐
☐
☐

If the sun is up while you're reading this, imagine that this evening is the last time that it will set. This is your last day. Mine as well. What should we do? How would you spend your time? We probably won't ever have the luxury of knowing the exact time of our deaths, but **thinking about it can help us reconnect with our priorities**.

If today were your last day, who would you be with? Who would you call on the phone? Where would you go? Would you be in a hurry? Would you want to relax in your favorite chair with a good book? What would you eat? What would you drink? Would food seem like a waste of time on today of all days, or would it be like saying goodbye to an old, favored friend?

You probably know where I'm going with this. It is possible to live everyday as if the stakes were that high.

Commitment: Live as if today is your last day. Do this every day. Because someday, you'll be right.

Journal...

_____
_____
_____
_____
_____
_____
_____
_____
_____
_____
_____
_____
_____
_____
_____
_____
_____
_____
_____
_____
_____
_____
_____

Thank you so much for purchasing this book!

Your purchase means a lot to me because it was made with your hard-earned money. I know you could've spent that money on other things. So I try to give you a lot of value for your dollar. Follow me on Facebook and Periscope so I can continue providing you with great content.

If this book has helped you, please leave me a review on Amazon.

About The Author

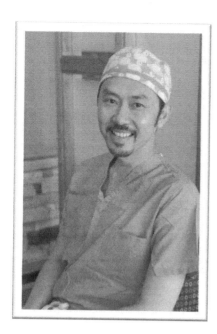

Dr. Duc Vuong is an internationally renowned bariatric surgeon, who is the world's leading expert in education for the bariatric patient. His intensive educational system has garnered attention from multiple institutions and medical societies. A prolific author, his passion in life is to fill the shortage of educational resources between patients and weight loss surgeons. Although trained in Western medicine, he blends traditional Eastern teachings with the latest in science and technology. Dr. Vuong was featured in TLC's hit show, 900 Pound Man: Race Against Time, and is currently working on his own weekly television show.

He currently works and lives in Albuquerque, NM. His daughter, Kizzie, has him wrapped around her little toe.

Visit Dr. Duc Vuong at www.UltimateGastricSleeve.com to learn more.

Other Books by Dr. Duc Vuong

Eating Healthy On A Budget: A How-To-Guide

Meditate to Lose Weight: A Guide For A Slimmer Healthier You

Healthy Green Smoothies: 50 Easy Recipes That Will Change Your Life

Big-Ass Salads: 31 Easy Recipes For Your Healthy Month

Love is Fishy: A Story of Romance and Recipes

Top 30 Exercise Myths for Weight Loss

Weight Loss Surgery Success: Dr. V's A-Z Steps For Losing Weight And Gaining Enlightenment

The Ultimate Gastric Sleeve Success: A Practical Patient Guide

Lap-Band Struggles: Revisit. Rethink. Revise.

Made in the USA
San Bernardino, CA
03 September 2016